Advance Praise for
Choosing to Die

A remarkable and sensitive portrayal of a family's journey with their mother to her assisted death, wrapped in the lore of Mom's garden plants, their cultivation, pleasure, and the wisdom of life's gifts. This book lifted me as a reader to profound new insights about life, death, grief, and bounteous love.

—Dr. Jean Marmoreo, CM, Co-author of *The Last Doctor: Lessons in Living from the Front Lines of Medical Assistance in Dying*

Evans' work is about the oldest subjects in existence—life, death, love, and family—and she ably navigates these turbulent waters, both as a writer and a daughter. She maintains a simple, clean prose style, even through the complicated decisions she had to make: "I feel nervous about making these decisions for Mom. Once again, my thoughts go to all the caregivers who are in the same spot as I am right now and have no medical background to support their decisions." Her straightforward style allows readers an unfiltered peek at intimate, trying moments.

A heartfelt chronicle of a family's reckoning with a complicated matriarch.

—*Kirkus Reviews*

Choosing to Die is Theresa Evans' inspirational and powerful exploration of her mother's choice to end her life using physician assistance.

She made the choice to die on her own terms, in her own home with her family at her side, creating beautiful memories up to the last day of her life.

As a geriatrician and certified hospice provider for over 20 years, I have seen firsthand the necessary components of "a good death."

Theresa takes us on a soulful journey with her family, using her mother's garden as a vibrant metaphor of life. She is exploring a topic which is uncomfortable for many, but in desperate need of being addressed with openness, honesty, and compassion.

Choosing to Die teaches us that all living beings who have managed to endure life's many ups and downs can find solace in knowing that with the proper plans in place, a "good death" is indeed possible.

—Peter Norvid, MD, Board certified in Geriatrics, Hospice and Palliative Care

I had planned to read Theresa's book gradually over the weekend, but once I started, I couldn't stop and was compelled to finish it in one sitting! What an outstanding celebration of life, of struggle, of overcoming, of love, of family, and finally of dying with one's dignity and grace well intact!

Theresa masterfully weaves together disparate themes—her mom's history, her own history, her mom's particular health issues, seen in the context of modern medicine and our current healthcare climate, her mom's garden and the family's collective love of plants, and the loving interaction between the sisters as they worked through anticipatory grief in the time leading up to her mom's death.

Forceful, irresistible, and gripping. I was caught up in the anticipation and suspense which the author brought to life and dispensed in such loving and well-crafted vignettes.

—John Clifford, M.D., Physical Medicine & Rehabilitation, MAiD Provider

Choosing to Die is a beautifully poignant story of love, loss, and legacy. Theresa Evans weaves the evolution of her mother's garden alongside the family's shared preparation for her mother's medically assisted death, using the changing seasons to guide us through their shared experience. Through thoughtful reflection, we are invited into her journey of profound loss and anticipatory grief, but also into the way her family remained deeply tethered to one another for support.

With profound honesty, Evans recognizes that time is both a gift and a burden, gracefully juxtaposing the desire for a loved one to be free from suffering with the heartache of not being ready to say goodbye. Yet, even in the darkness, there is a steady sense of light and meaning found in each remaining moment. Together, they find ways to honor their mother and each other through the living legacy of her garden, shared and carried forward with love.

—Kim Carlson and Paul Magennis, Registered Nurses and MAiD Educators, authors of Substack *MAiD in Canada*

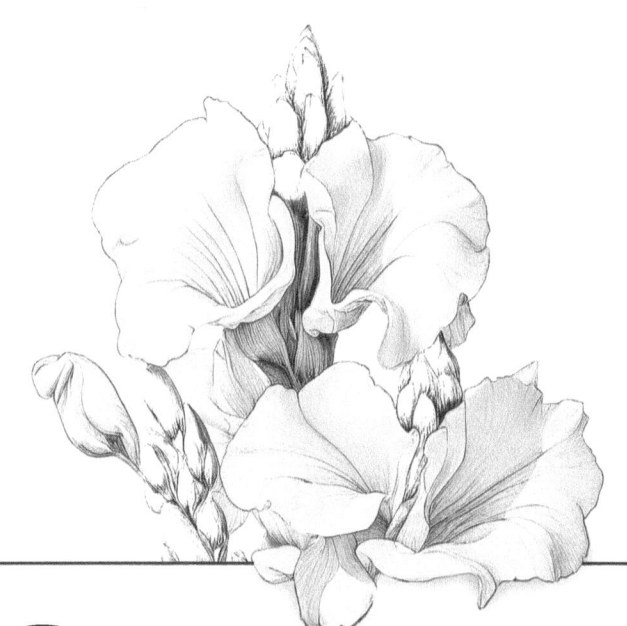

Choosing to Die

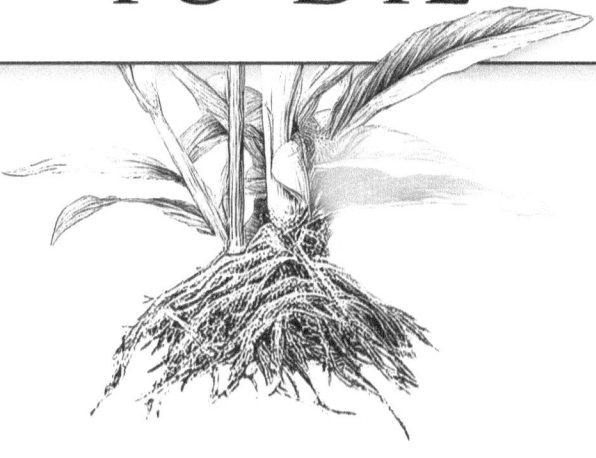

A Daughter's Story Of
Supporting Her Mother's End
Of Life Through Assisted Death

Theresa E. Evans

Copyright © 2025 Theresa E. Evans
ALL RIGHTS RESERVED
Some names have been changed to protect the identities of survivors, friends, and family. The conversations, details, dates, and the sequences of events contained in this book are relayed to the best of my knowledge and ability. Some dialogue has been re-created in some conversations.

No part of this book may be translated, used, or reproduced in any form or by any means, in whole or in part, electronic or mechanical, including photocopying, recording, taping, or by any information storage or retrieval system without express written permission from the author or the publisher, except for the use in brief quotations within critical articles and reviews.

Theresa.e.evans@gmail.com

Limits of Liability and Disclaimer of Warranty:
The authors and/or publisher shall not be liable for your misuse of this material. The contents are strictly for informational and educational purposes only.

Warning/Disclaimer

The information provided about assisted death (also known as medical aid in dying or physician-assisted dying) is for informational and educational purposes only. This information should not be taken as medical or legal advice. It is crucial to consult with qualified healthcare professionals and legal experts for specific guidance on individual situations related to end-of-life care and choices, especially for those considering assisted death.

The author and/or publisher do not guarantee that anyone following these techniques, suggestions, tips, ideas, or strategies will become successful. The author and/or publisher shall have neither liability nor responsibility to anyone with respect to any loss or damage caused, or alleged to be caused, directly or indirectly by the information contained in this book. Further, readers should be aware that Internet websites listed in this work may have changed or disappeared between when this work was written and when it is read.

Printed and bound in the United States of America
ISBNs:
Hardback: 979-8-9932663-0-5
Paperback: 979-8-9932663-3-6
Ebook: 979-8-9932663-1-2
Audiobook: 979-8-9932663-2-9

For Mom,
who taught me the art of
daughtering...
&
For Stephanie,
who is teaching me the art of
mothering.

After her death, I found this list among my mother's papers.

> Choices in life
> Having children
> stop having children
> Getting Married
> divorce
> Many Life choices Big + sm.
> Choosing to die
>
> check Life ins.
>
> Clear your soul
>
> Clear my conscience

Contents

Preface 1
Introduction 5

PART I: SUMMER'S END 13
   Chapter 1: Mom's Garden 15
   Chapter 2: Anemones 25
   Chapter 3: Snapdragons 41
   Chapter 4: Water Lilies 57

PART II: AUTUMN'S GIFTS 73
   Chapter 5: Moonflower 75
   Chapter 6: Cosmos 91
   Chapter 7: Purple Coneflower 123
   Chapter 8: Foxglove 137
   Chapter 9: Asters 149
   Chapter 10: Roses 161
   Chapter 11: Lavender 175
   Chapter 12: Sedum 185
   Chapter 13: Christmas Cactus 197

PART III: WINTER'S APPROACH 207
   Chapter 14: Sugar Maple Tree 209
   Chapter 15: Fly to the Light 245

Epilogue: Grief 257
Author's Note 265
Resources 269
Acknowledgments 271
Glossary 273
About the Author 279

Preface

My mom is drowning. Coarse wet rattles announce her inhalations, followed by incomplete and ineffective impostors posing as exhalations. Her hazel-gray eyes glisten as they fix on mine, and we spill into each other the way mothers and daughters sometimes do. An enduring contract sealed with our shared DNA has lasted a lifetime; the bounty of stored memories now and then blurs who is the mother and who is the daughter. Her eyes plead with me to *make. this. stop.* "*You can do it, Theresa. You can do anything you set your mind to. I've watched you do it your whole life, dear...*" I scream a silent protest, "*But I don't want to be the oldest daughter right now, Mom...*"

I know there is no amount of *setting my mind to it* that can repair her tired and broken heart. I only know one way to *make. this. stop*, but now is not the time for a life-and-death conversation. Something that rarely happens when the living is easy. *Who wants to spoil a good life by talking about death?* Any prospects of being thrown a life jacket vanish when together we decide *not* to call 911. *Now, we're really "in it."* I give Mom some of the liquid gold narcotic that will dilate her veins and arteries and lessen the burden of breathing for the moment.

A thief tries to steal my breath with a tightening that grips the center of my chest. I won't give him a second chance. *One of us has to keep breathing.* I am desperate to ease Mom's suffering, but I can't let my desperation distract me from focusing. Summoning up all my courage, I crawl into bed with Mom. There is nothing easy about this moment. It takes more effort than it should to slide Mom up the wall to an upright position that helps her breathe. She leans her sticky, sweat-soaked back into my front. Her heart is too big and the muscle is too weak. Like a drummer who has lost the rhythm, the beats fire randomly and ineffectively; they collide with my fear. *My* heart wants to beat for her, but right now it feels tenuous and unkempt. It's time to let my *nurse brain* take over for long enough to form a plan.

I can smell the *old* version of Mom, part of the chemical and hormonal changes that accompany

Preface

aging. Despite our culture's best attempts and frequent claims, we have not yet managed to reverse this process. Quietly, I am coaching her through each breath as my cells are viscerally imagining my life without her. When she starts talking to people I can't see, my nurse brain registers this as further evidence that she is flirting with life or dancing with death. *It could go either way.* Together we have slid down in the bed. The front of my knees are tucked into the back of her knees. *We are spooning like lovers.* If she is leaving, I want to feel her leave. I want her spirit to flow through me like electricity on its way out of her body. I want her to imprint all of her mother-love into my cells. I learn it is possible to hold dread and wonder at the same time.

We are wrapped in a veil of silence. The persistent whirring of the oxygen machine that sounded so invasive thirty minutes ago has now become white noise. My chest feels the barely perceptible rising and falling of her chest. The morphine is working. She has drifted into sleep. I close my eyes and breathe for both of us. *It will be four more years before I lie down with my mom and she leaves her body.*

Choosing to die

Introduction

Journal entry August 21, 2020. *After two weeks in quarantine due to Covid, I am relieved to have moved into Mom's home and settled in for the next three months. She has chosen her 80th birthday to drop her body. The rich palette of the summer is on full display in Mom's garden. Sun glints off abundant shades of greens and illuminates the flowers in a kaleidoscope of color; boundaries are muddled as one plant spills into another. Bees unwittingly carry the pollen collected on their hairy bodies from plant to plant; butterflies flit amongst the flowers, seeking out their soft landings, and droplets of water twirl in the air as songbirds bathe in the pond to clean their feathers. It is still the season of activity and growth.*

Despite the cacophony of life and color surrounding me, a heavy, dull ache has taken root in my sternum. This is the last season I will stand in my mother's garden. In eighty-six days, she will lie down and she will not get up. Right now, eighty-six days feels like enough, but I know time will warp my perception, and eighty-six days will feel like eighty-six minutes. This entry is the beginning of a journal I will keep to document these last days with Mom and my sisters. Eighty-six days until November 15.

Mom has chosen to die on November 15 at 11:00 a.m. *Medical Assistance in Dying,* or *MAID,* has been legal in Canada since 2016. By 2023, 60,301 Canadians had died using MAID. We have heard the objections of those who consider this an abomination: a sin against God and a selfish decision that is not ours to make. These religious and philosophical objections have prompted Mom to keep her decision to a close circle of family and friends. It is enough to consciously die; *for even when death feels like a welcome reprieve, we are hardwired to live.* Once the choice has been made, there is no room for the opinions of others. Her body, mind, and heart must meld into a cohesive unit in support of this literal life-altering decision.

This is but one of the ethical dilemmas we find ourselves divided over in our current culture. Resolving

INTRODUCTION

these dilemmas is not the purpose of this book. I am not writing to take on these big questions. I am writing to record the final days spent with my mom before she lay down in her bed and received the medication that stopped her breathing and ended her life. I am writing for myself as I continue the process of integrating and accepting that she *really is gone*. I am writing for my daughter Stephanie, who was not able to be with us. I am writing for anyone who has thought about medically assisted death as an option, and I am writing for those who have *never* considered medically assisted death as an option. Before this, I would have put giving birth to my daughter at the top of my list of *most profound life experiences*. Now a birth and a death share equal weight in my heart. So, I write because I feel called to share this most profound experience with anyone who feels called to read about it.

For four years before Mom's death, I made multiple emergency visits home. There is never a convenient time to be called to your mother's deathbed. Our lives are filled with countless moving parts, and mine is no exception. These twelve-hour drives were arduous. I vacillated between *guilt* and *envy* that my younger sisters were there shouldering the hands-on care. I had moved a thousand miles away in my late teens. Now in my late fifties, I was scheming ways to return to my family's hometown in southwestern Ontario. Autopilot got me through these long drives home. Years of navigating this trip made my internal GPS more reliable than my current muddled mind and my tear-filled vision.

Emanating from deep beneath the surface of my breastbone was a hot and heavy sensation. This is where the ache of getting there too late to say goodbye and hold Mom one last time always took up residence. And what if she didn't die? Would this be but one more step deeper into the downward spiral that had become her current quality of life? The medications and interventions promising relief from the ravages of end-stage heart failure and chronic obstructive pulmonary disease (COPD) felt like broken promises. When did my prayers shift from wanting her to live? Now I prayed that these interventions tenuously tethering Mom to her physical body would prove ineffective. That the power of her free spirit would take flight. More than anything, I wanted Mom to

Introduction

die peacefully. I prayed that if grace and the universe were on my side, I would be there with her when she left.

I had memorized my way through the maze of elevators and long corridors in this hospital hundreds of miles from my home. I knew which floor the ICU was on as my hand automatically reached for the buzzer to ask for admittance. I knew which floor the cafeteria was on. I knew where to park without having to pay. I knew how to navigate the after-hours entrance.

Like entering a church, I quietly tiptoed into the ICU. Instead of an altar, there was the nurse's station. The hub of the unit. As a registered nurse, I had spent several years working in Intensive Care Units. I knew the protocol. I knew how to approach without being labeled a needy family member. Bowing and making the sign of the cross were replaced with a nod and a glance. Tithing included a box of bagels for the nurses. Time and circumstances would dictate whether I felt the need to flex my *nursing muscle* to advocate for Mom. My heart belonged to the child who loved her mother. My brain had been taught to make meaningful medical decisions.

It was always the middle of the night when I arrived. My sisters would ask me to wait until morning. Common sense told me to wait until morning, but I was never willing to hedge my bet that Mom would still be there if I delayed my arrival by even a few hours. On one of these visits, I walked into Mom's room after completing a ten-hour drive not knowing whether she was dead or alive. This was before the days of cell phones. I wrapped my arms around her and held her close. I told her how glad I was that she was still alive so I could tell her how much I loved her. Years later, she would tell me, "That was the moment I knew you really loved me." Mom and I shared a complicated kind of love.

It was a relief when she was admitted to the intensive care unit. The alternative was a ward or a shared room. This is Canada, where most hospitals are utilitarian and not five-star hotels. The ICU meant a private room filled with silence, save for the beeps and humming of the monitors recording vital signs for the doctors and nurses. I watched her sleep. The hospital gown and bedsheets were tangled around her. Mom's knees were drawn up toward her chin while her shoulders and head curled down toward

INTRODUCTION

her knees. I recognized this protective posture; the fetal position is the oldest hardwired reflex in all living creatures. We spend our first nine months in the womb in this position. I have heard it said those nine months are our most peaceful and where we feel the safest. Whenever we feel threatened, an unconscious response activates and curls us into versions of this round ball. We do it to protect our vital organs. We do it to protect our heart. We all do it—even woolly caterpillars do it. Mom was imitating a woolly caterpillar while her nervous system responded to pain and fear.

Even with the oxygen face mask, her breaths were shallow. She looked worn-out, tired and fragile. When she opened her eyes, they glistened not with life, but with fear. Silently, Mom was pleading with me to help her. Despite my years as a registered nurse, I felt completely inept. *Did she want me to help her live or did she want me to help her die?*

CHOOSING TO DIE

Part One
SUMMER'S END

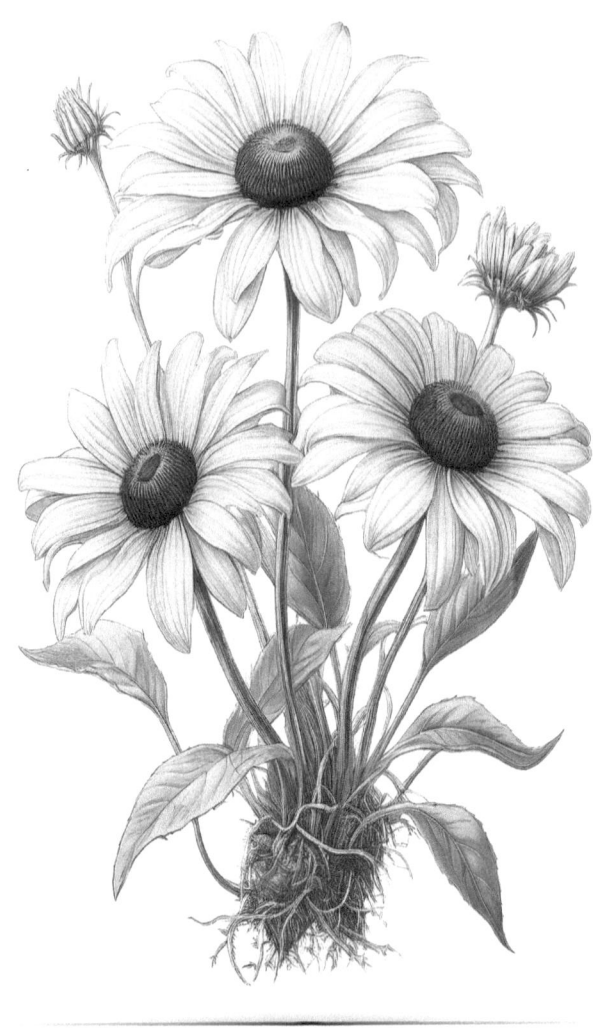

Rudbeckia hirta
Common Name – Black-Eyed Susan

*Like the plants in Mom's garden,
for everything there is a life cycle.*

Chapter One

Mom's Garden

Journal entry August 25, 2020. Today the weather is warm and sunny, and I look forward to time in the garden. Mom's garden has been her refuge, and now it will be mine. I will resist the urge to coddle Mom and grow my sensitivity around her needs. Eighty-two days until November 15.

In my mother's wild and effusive flower garden, hardy clumps of *Rudbeckia* live up to their common name of black-eyed Susans. Staring back at me with their brown-black pistils, they mirror my own dark pupils. Golden petals compete for space with wild recklessness. They stand in stark contrast to the tall purple, orderly, regal liatris, giving the illusion the fence is merely for decoration and not a true boundary. Butter-yellow snapdragons poke their heads through the white pickets.

Closing my eyes, I place my hand over my breastbone. I learned to call this area my *heart center* when I taught yoga. I want to feel this ache whose weight keeps me present. I am standing in *Tadasana* or Mountain Pose. Years and hours spent practicing on my yoga mat show up to support my intention to stay grounded. In this foundational pose my hand becomes a lightning rod and my nervous system becomes the grounding wire as I direct my fear, sadness, and confusion through my feet and into the earth. My heart is fragile. I need to titrate these emotions. It is too much to feel all at once. I don't want to miss the *mystery* of Mom's leaving. The solid ground beneath my feet will support this journey.

Like a rough, thick tuber storing nutrients for the plant underground, my heart has stored a lifetime of memories that bind me to my family. While the *details* of our memories are influenced by context, past events, and time, the *emotion*s connected to those memories often lie closer to the surface and feel easier to recall.

Note: You'll find a glossary of gardening words and terms in the back of this book.

Chapter One: Mom's Garden

Our memories vary depending on who in the family is telling the story. I consider my youngest sister to be the *memory keeper* for our family. She remembers the details that I forgot I lived. While I have always *lived big,* she has lived *meticulously.* Both ways have their unique blessings and curses. My middle sister came in with Mom's strong psychic abilities and connection to energy patterns. More than once, I have benefited from her powerful Reiki. The beauty of Mom's garden is reflected in the variety of flora and fauna. This is the same for families.

There are times when the environment changes and doesn't support growth. There may be too many plants competing for too few nutrients and not enough sunlight; this was the case in my mom's biological family when they immigrated to Canada in the 1930s. These stressors can be remedied by thinning the plants *or by giving your two youngest children away.* Amending the soil, careful watering, and attention to light sources may be necessary. It's the same for all gardens and for most families.

Research shows the strong connection between how loved we felt as a child and how we are able to manage difficult experiences as an adult. I have stored many stories of Mom's harsh childhood as the second youngest of eight siblings. Her parents immigrated from Ireland to Toronto, Ontario, with nothing but the clothes on their backs in search of a better life. That dream was confiscated by alcohol and petty crime. My maternal grandfather spent most of his life in and out of jail for these offenses until he was literally escorted out of town and told never to return. My grandmother felt she had no choice but to surrender my mother and Mom's youngest sister to the Ontario Children's Aid Society.

Even though these amendments will support growth and vitality, they can be shocking at first. Plant shock occurs as a result of environmental stressors: too much or too little water, too much or too little sunlight, drastic temperature changes or overfertilization. During this period of adjustment, leaves may appear wilted, discolored, or even fall to the ground; the flower may not bloom, the bloom might be delayed or uncharacteristically small, and the plant may lack vitality. It takes time for a plant to acclimate to changes. This timing is also true with families.

Chapter One: Mom's Garden

Mom made it to the fifth grade in school but spent most of her childhood caring for other people's children, cooking, and cleaning other people's homes. Her lack of education and a nurturing environment lit a fire in her to be a good mother and a good wife. To create a happy home. Unfortunately, neither she nor my father had any actual experience living in a stable home. They were both only seventeen years young when they had their first child.

I notice there are weeds in Mom's garden that she has not been able to pull. Weeds grow in all gardens; what one gardener considers a weed, another considers a medicinal treasure. My sisters and I will pull the weeds for Mom. We have been doing this since we were young. This is *why* we are able to gather now—my sisters, my mother, and me. We have been tending the family garden for years. We can support each other in Mom's decision to die.

There are processes taking place out of sight in all gardens and I suspect in all families. Newly spawned offspring tubers buried in the earth will grow shoots in the spring, and these shoots will produce stems and leaves for the coming season. *Degeneration* and *regeneration* carry the same weight in nature.

They complement each other. One cannot succeed without the other. It appears we are not designed to live in our physical bodies forever. Like the plants in Mom's garden, for everything there is a life cycle.

The lifespan for plants is determined genetically. Annuals live for one year, biennials live for two years, and perennials can live indefinitely. These life cycles are tied to the seasons, particularly light and temperature. Plants also need water and oxygen. For humans, the life cycle is determined by lifestyle, environment, and genetics. Genetics have the least influence—around twenty to thirty percent of a person's lifespan. In the summer, tubers from last season will decay and new tubers will begin to grow. Right now, the tuber that occupies my heart feels rough and scaly and shriveled, and *that feels right for the season of letting go.*

Reverence and gratitude wash over me as I gather Mom's garden tools. These tools have become an extension of her hands over the years. They are old and well-used. She has her favorites, but none are fancy. The long, serrated bread knife can separate bulbs and aerate a root ball just as well as it can slice bread for dinner. Mom has asked me to do this

Chapter One: Mom's Garden

annual rite of fall for her. To tend to her most precious space. *She must trust me.* Something that takes a lifetime to build, trust has been given and taken and given again in our years of raising each other.

I see her gazing through the open window from her chair. She is energetically pulling at me with a powerful call that does not rely on words. I feel her ache to join me—to dig her hands into the rich soil she has been cultivating. To smell the last lingering fragrances of the flowers' perfumes mingled with the earthier scents of humus being carried away on the wind. She longs to take in the textures and colors, not through a pane of glass but sensorily by touch and scent. She wants to give me one last tip to carry home to my own garden.

Late summer lilacs make themselves known as their distinct sweet aroma fills my nostrils. I wonder if these lilacs are designed to bloom this late or if they are here to say goodbye like I am. I feel the weight of getting this done exactly the way Mom herself would do it if she was able. I start to regret not taking full advantage of the gardening knowledge she has learned from minutes and hours and years spent with her hands covered in earth. She has been listening to the secrets the plants whispered. *Plants have always been more reliable than people in Mom's life.*

When Mom bought this bland tiny square house on a slightly run-down street, in a more than slightly run-down city, I voiced my concern, "There is no room for your garden, Mom. The soil is mostly clay and dry, a hostile environment for a garden ..." But she was steadfast in her conviction that this was the house. A place where she could heal and create a home. This same determination fueled Mom's longing to grow a family, the family she had longed for as a child. Remember, *what one gardener considers a weed, another gardener sees as medicinal bounty.* Mom took the foundation of weeds she had been raised on, and with all the care she could muster, she began to plant flowers in her garden literally and figuratively to nourish her family.

Chapter One: Mom's Garden

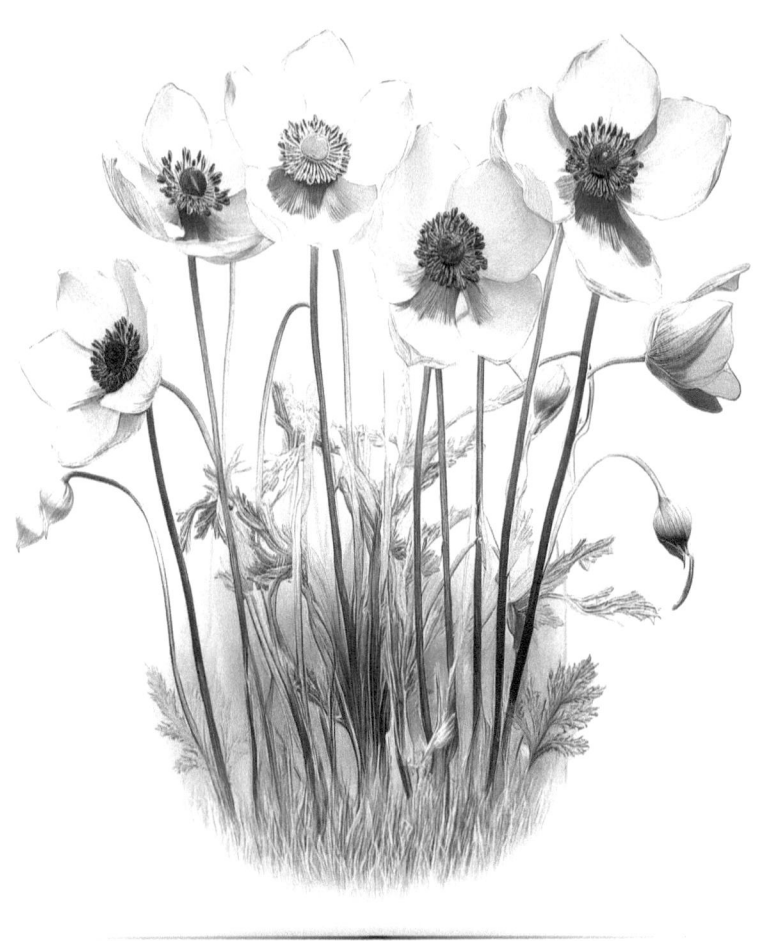

Ranunculaceae

Common Name – Anemones

They stand strong on their own, scramble to find their place in the group as the winds change.... This is the same rhythm my sisters and I are dancing to right now.

Chapter Two

ANEMONES

Journal entry August 30, 2020. *It is a very raw time for all of us. Filled with the most sweet and tender moments, along with the darker shadow moments when old family patterns arise. So old—perhaps carried down in our genes by the genes of our ancestors. But we are all in and committed to being present for Mom's passing. We are entering the season of letting go where seeds fall, leaves drop, and mothers prepare to die. Seventy-seven days until November 15.*

My gaze settles on the large patch of anemones in Mom's garden. These delicate, pure white flowers have five fragile petals that together form a corolla the size of a silver dollar. Bright fuzzy lemon-yellow stamens join into perfectly round circles, as if drawn with nature's protractor. They grace the center of each corolla. Like nimble dancers, their long green gangly stems surrender to the urgings of the late summer breeze. The origin story of anemones is found in Greek mythology. When Aphrodite's lover Adonis is killed by a wild boar while hunting, it is said her tears mixed with the blood of her lover, and wherever they fell to the earth, red anemones bloomed. Red and pink anemones symbolize death, grief, and abandoned love. Mom's delicate white anemones are a symbol of sincerity.

These anemones are every bit of four feet tall. They stand strong on their own, scramble to find their place in the group as the winds change, and then settle into the quiet of the moment. This is the same rhythm my sisters and I are dancing to right now. There is so much raw emotion we are feeling individually and collectively. After many years of living apart, we have come together at this vulnerable, raw, and most significant time. Old emotions surface and long-forgotten memories of wounds that have never been voiced hover precariously at the edges of our psyches.

Today started out tough. Events occurred which are not even important to remember. What *is* import-

Chapter Two: Anemones

ant is that we all stayed and showed up. My sisters, my mom, and I sat in four corners of the living room at an impasse. "If you girls don't get along and straighten this out, I am going to call the doctor and move everything up to this week," declared Mom. I looked at her—actually I glared at her. OK ... all cards were on the table. "You can't threaten us with your assisted death, Mom."

I got up and walked down the stairs to my room feeling utterly distraught. My sisters went home, and Mom collapsed onto her bed. We left each other in a very sad, quiet way. I felt stuck. Truthfully, I considered leaving. I asked myself, *"What would that feel like?"* Then I asked myself, *"What would it feel like to stay ... even if staying feels like being crushed?"* The second option still felt better, even if it involved a bit of crushing. I had already lived out the first option. The tears started flowing and I let myself feel it all. I let the tears wash away my hardness. Then I texted my sisters ...

Me: "That was really hard, sisters."
Sister #1: "Really, really hard. I feel very sad."
Sister #2: "Same."
Me: "Me too. I feel broken."

Sister #2: "Same. I'm open to anything to heal this."

Sister #1: "Well, that makes three of us."

Me: "Well, maybe it's safer for us from a distance right now. To feel a little softer toward all of us. I'm struggling with Mom's threat."

Sister #2: "I really don't want us to break up."

Me: "This shit is what drove me away the first time."

Sister #1: "I'm struggling with that as well. I feel it's not safe to feel."

Me: "I don't want us to break up either. That's a very sad option. This is some of the really hard clearing we are being asked to do right now, that can only be done in the midst of this kind of really deep energy."

Sister #2: "I think if we think of it as less of a threat and more of a 'what can she do to help us get through this in one piece?' I'm not trying to make an excuse for her, but she's going someplace she has no idea about and leaving us behind."

Me: "She really triggered all of my hardness toward her. I was fourteen years old again in that room with Mom telling me to shape up or get out ... Feels familiar."

Sister #1: "I do get what you are saying."

Me: "I'm in a dark place that I thought was cleared."

Sister #1: "Do you want to come over?"

Chapter Two: Anemones

Sister #2: "Mom has been and is going to be a very hard teacher right until the end."

Me: "Yes."

Sister #1: "Do you want to walk?"

Sister #2: "Is Mom up?"

Me: "I can't stop crying. We could walk, but it needs to be all of us."

Sister #1: "I'm crying too."

Sister #2: "Let's meet at (my sister's place). I'll leave now."

Sister #1: "OK."

Me: "Mom's in bed but possibly awake."

Sister #1: "Just let her know you are going for a walk."

Me: "We should wake her up for a group cry-hug."

Sister #2: "OK. I'm sure she's feeling it too. Let's meet at Mom's."

Me "We just need to feel we can all show up soft and safe. I'll wait for you guys."

Sister #1: "OK."

I didn't realize I had written this conversation out exactly the way I have written it here. I found it in a separate journal during the writing of this book. There are moments when words feel insufficient. This was one of those moments. We came together and wrapped our arms around each other and connected with our hearts. I will be forever grateful we all chose to come back together. We held each other. We shed rivers of tears. We went into Mom's room and woke her up so she was included in this group hug that would set the tone for the rest of our time together. If we were moving ourselves into the brightest, lightest version of ourselves, we had to acknowledge all of it.

I watch hundreds of sun-yellow discs in white circle skirts sway like a choir as Claude Debussy's Arabesque No. 1 plays in my head. Years of piano lessons have become the musical backdrop for nature's spontaneous dance recital. When you look at a plant, you only see half of it, or sometimes less than half. The rest is buried below the surface and out of sight. Music was a seed Mom had stored since her childhood. Early in our elementary-school years, she asked each of us to choose a musical instrument to study.

A family struggling to meet the basic needs of food, clothing, and shelter does not consider piano

CHAPTER TWO: ANEMONES

lessons a viable option. Mom's longing lay dormant in a seed full of potential buried deep in her psyche. Some of us garden for the flowers. The beauty we see on the surface. Some of us are drawn to the science of gardening and the mysteries held by the seeds and germination. You can't have one without the other. From the perspective of the plant, the sole purpose of the flower is to attract pollinators to move the pollen from the anther to the stigma to fertilize the fruit that will bear the seeds. It's all about ensuring continuation of the species.

Mom took a job in a factory to purchase my piano and pay for my lessons. This is a great weight to carry as a child ... *knowing your mom has gone to work to pay for your piano lessons.* I have always loved music—listening to it, playing it, even dabbling with writing it—and I am forever grateful for my years of lessons. *That which we can see* became clear when my natural talent and strong determination resulted in my scoring the second highest mark in Ontario after taking the yearly conservatory exam.

Mom has asked me to dig up a large clump of anemones for the minister who is coming to visit this afternoon. They are crowded together, and their long stems tangle easily. Digging up a clump without disturbing the petals or breaking the stems proves challenging. The roots are crowded and firmly anchored in their earthen home. I should cut down the stems and flowers and deliver a healthy root ball ... but an old story is driving me to retain the *beauty we can see*.

    I would receive my silver medal at a recital where all of the top scorers were slated to play. I practiced my piece. I memorized it. I played it a thousand times. I played it on the dining-room table. I played it on my desk at school. I played it in my dreams. In a large hall on a gleaming grand piano on a stage in front of my mother, my teacher, and all those attending, my joy began to dim. Weeds appeared in the midst of the stanzas. Being the *keeper of the music* for our family felt like too great a responsibility. Fear that I could not bloom bright enough marred my performance. I barely remember it. What I do remember is feeling I had let Mom down. I don't remember ever seeing that damn silver medal. I asked Mom about it recently and she has no idea what might have happened to it. I cut back the anemones and dig up a robust and healthy root ball. With the right soil and water, *that*

Chapter Two: Anemones

which we cannot see will support that which we can see in the spring.

I play the guitar and the hammered dulcimer these days. I taught myself. I picked up these instruments because Mom planted a seed when I was young. She loves to hear me play. Sometimes you think you have culled a plant from the garden, only to find a shoot has been slowly germinating underground. *When that which we cannot see supports that which we can see.*

Vast and clear and robin's egg blue is the fall sky. "This would be a good day to take flight, Mom … clear skies ahead." I smile at this youthful version of what happens when we die. As if Mom is going to magically fly up and enter the six-year-old version of heaven I had imagined and stored during my elementary years. In their black-and-white habits, the gatekeepers of the Father, the Son, and the Holy Ghost drip-fed eight years of catechism into my young mind. Like roots storing nutrients for the plant, my mind stored the concrete images of heaven and hell taught by the nuns at Holy Rosary Elementary School. Mom embraced the Roman Catholic doctrine with a fervor known only by those who have lived abandonment, felt alone, and held tight to anything close to belonging. The Bible with its gold edges and frightening pictures set me on a path I would explore for the rest of my life, *a more compassionate possibility for heaven and hell.*

Closing my eyes, I inhale the scent of the lake carried on the winds. Lake Erie is only eight miles from here. The sandy shores of the shallowest Great Lake were our playgrounds as children. To this day, my soul feels thirsty when I am away from water for an extended period of time. Mom is craving fish and chips, so we have planned a day trip to the local beach we frequented as children. We are all reveling in the light following our hard conversation in the morning. *This is how it will be, I think; moments of light will intersperse with moments of dark.* Our hearts will show up like dappled sunlight.

I remember well the cacophony of activity involved in loading the car with four kids—*three girls and a boy*—soaked in suntan lotion, with yellow plastic shovels, old ice cream buckets for sandcastles, striped towels, and coolers filled with sandwiches and drinks. In contrast, this trip will require two full

Chapter Two: Anemones

portable oxygen tanks, nitroglycerin in case of chest pain, an emergency inhaler, something for anxiety, and a cane or a walker.

Our mother-daughter roles have reversed and feel topsy-turvy, like the leaves scattered about the garden. They are still green, but they have left the mother tree early. I have given up trying to rake them into a pile; they are under the spell of the capricious winds. Every task I take on presents itself like practice for the final moment with Mom. For a person who has spent a good deal of her life attempting to create order out of chaos, I now feel completely out of my element. *There's no controlling something I can't even fathom.*

Mom has a phone call scheduled with Sister Mary Catherine, who started visiting during Mom's frequent hospitalizations. "Why, Mom? You know she will not support your decision. It's against the laws of the church." Mom answers without wavering that if Sister Mary Catherine can talk her out of the MAID program, she should not be going through with it. This is a test to see if her conviction is strong and her reasoning sound. She has long ago separated her relationship with God from the institution of the church. I admire my mom deeply in this moment and I rest in her power.

She has shown me three rosaries. My mother's devotion to the Catholic Church has waxed and waned over the years, but she has never wavered in her commitment to God, Mother Teresa, and the Rosary. One of her most prized possessions is a letter signed by Mother Teresa thanking Mom for spearheading a campaign that sent hundreds of rosaries to Calcutta in support of Mother Teresa's work. As children, my sisters and I wore an indentation into the hardwood floors with our knees. Praying the Rosary happened every night for years in our home. We prayed before meals, giving thanks for our bounty. We prayed before sleep, that we might wake in the morning. We prayed as atonement for guileless childhood sins we had committed. We prayed to celebrate happenings in the present moment and prayed for something that could create a brighter future ... like world peace. It seemed no ask was too great if prayed with the appropriate reverence and humility.

This future tense bit confused me as a child. Didn't one of the Ten Commandments ask us not to covet, not to lust after things? World peace felt

Chapter Two: Anemones

like a big ask, even to me. As a child praying the Rosary, my thoughts hovered between preoccupation with my sore knees, fear that I *really could* be struck by lightning, and counting ahead with a free finger to determine how many more decades were on the rosary before we were finished. I know how hard it would have been for Mom to even consider entering the MAID program if she had any inclination it would be a sin against God. Mom had shared with us that after minutes and hours and days and nights of prayer, she felt clear with God. Her health issues were man-made and not God-made. Man's interventions were keeping her alive, and man's interventions would end this cycle. God was waiting for her.

These days I think of the rosary as a Catholic-inspired *mala*. A tool I can use to grow more awareness and intention in *my* life. Each of these three rosaries holds a place of devotion and love in Mom's heart. She has been praying them for years. She keeps them in a silk pouch hidden under her pillow. One rosary for each of her living daughters—Mom's reassurance to us that we will always be connected. I treasure my rosary. I feel Mom's energy when I hold it. Sometimes I say the traditional Rosary and sometimes I simply hold it, passing each bead through my fingers while talking to Mom.

Wetting the earthen ball of roots that supports the anemones, I wrap it in newspaper and place it in a bag. Despite my digging, the anemones look none the worse for wear. They are resilient. A metaphor for a life well-lived. If you Google the word "resilient," it is described as "an individual's ability to successfully adapt to life tasks in the face of social disadvantage or highly adverse conditions." I have watched Mom grow her capacity for resilience my entire life. As her heart has grown weaker, she has struggled to slowly surrender her independence. Despite her early childhood years, Mom has always managed to actively participate in creating a life that worked for her. Sometimes at great mental, emotional, and physical cost to herself and those around her. I look up and see the minister walking down the street.

Chapter Two: Anemones

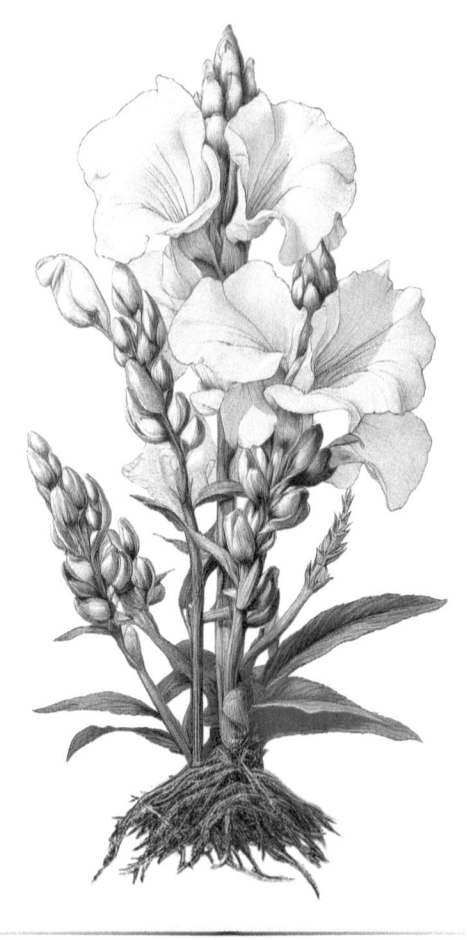

Antirrhinum majus
Common Name – Snapdragons

Snapdragons are some of the last bloomers to die off. Mom's health has imitated these snapdragons by bouncing back again and again and again when we thought she could not, when we were told she would not.

Chapter Three

SNAPDRAGONS

Journal entry September 8, 2020. *Yesterday, I found the Mother's Day card I had sent to Mom in May. It was tucked into one of the many stacks of important papers that fill the tables in her living room. It appeared like a buried treasure, reminding me of how I have been preparing for this moment for some time now. May is when we began talking about the MAID program and Mom was starting to feel it could be the right choice for her. Sixty-eight days until November 15.*

Back then I was calling Mom every day, even though my work schedule of frequent domestic and international travel made it challenging. I would often bring home greeting cards created by local artists bought in quaint owner-operated galleries. This beautiful color lithograph card was not an *actual* Mother's Day card, but my heart chose it. It would be the last card I would send to Mom to mark this day that celebrates mothers.

A young girl stands on a tall branch in a towering white pine tree. One hand grasps the tree, while her other hand holds a walking stick. Her long blond hair is being tousled by the wind. Her red skirt swirls around her ankles, and the sleeves of her white blouse are rolled up as if to ready herself for the task at hand. She wears a backpack. Her bare feet stand strong on the tree branch and belie the precariousness of her perch. Her presence conjures up a sense of strength and mystery, as she gazes off into the horizon.

On one branch sits an owl with piercing round eyes. The owl is watching a medium-sized black bear climb the tree. The bear is not menacing, but rather curious as it peers out into the same vast horizon as the girl. Another branch holds a crow whose face is turned away from the bear. The words at the top of the card read *"From a Great Height, She Saw What Could Be Seen."* The card is blank inside. My message reads …

Chapter Three: Snapdragons

Dear Mom,

This may seem like a strange Mother's Day card, but the girl in the tree reminds me of you. She's you with your backpack on, getting ready to take your next great adventure. "She came to visit, she stayed awhile, and then it was time to leave." This is what you have been telling me. Look at the strong bear totem in the tree. The bear represents the depth of power that you possess. The bear is also about patience and perfect timing. The crow in the tree symbolizes the magic and mysteries that exist in our lives. The crow means you should leave all the past behind you as something new is being born. And the girl also represents me. Your oldest living daughter. I stand in the tree on this strong branch of wisdom and shout out how much I love you. I am aware you are transforming, and I treasure every moment we still share together. Thank you for showing up for this mother-daughter journey. It's not always easy and it is also magical. One of our most important relationships. Love you so much, Mom, xo Theresa

Antirrhinum majus or snapdragons are *my* favorite garden flower. They have always made a showy splash of color in Mom's gardens with their saturated hues of deep red and purple in contrast to the pastel yellows, whites, and shades of pink. Mom's snapdragons are predominantly yellow, the color symbolizing joy and happiness. Perfect. We can still know joy; we can still *be* joy in the midst of Mom's transition. Their sturdy tall stems are considered a symbol of strength. I will pick a bouquet for all of us and let the snapdragons energetically surround us with these qualities.

Specifically associated with feminine strength, respect, and grace, snapdragons can grow in rocky ground that sometimes appears to lack soil. They can endure extreme conditions and a variety of temperatures, including a light frost. Folklore tells us that when a man gives a woman a gift of snapdragons, they convey his love and respect for her strength. *There is that which we can see and that which we cannot see.* While a plant may appear to be growing in rocks, the roots have actually anchored in the bits of soil hidden between and beneath the rocks. Even rock gardens require some soil.

This was true for Mom. Despite her stories of a childhood marred by too little love and too much

Chapter Three: Snapdragons

suffering, she managed to take root and receive *enough* nutrients in *enough* soil to grow. A plant may not *thrive* in less-than-ideal conditions, but many are remarkably resilient—especially the part *which we cannot see.* Mom's early memories are fractured and blur between stretches in foster homes and stints with her birth family. She remembers being molested in her crib as a toddler. She remembers living in one run-down room with her parents and seven other siblings. She remembers the only bathroom was in the hallway. She remembers old men she didn't know watch her use that toilet because the shared bathroom had no door. She remembers being hungry. She remembers sleeping on benches in the park. She remembers being cold. She remembers her father trying to sell her. *So much hard clay soil.*

Just when root rot might have set in, my grandmother's mother-love took over and she moved her plant to what she hoped would be a permanent location. She gave Mom to a young couple who had not been able to conceive a child of their own. Mom lived with this couple long enough to believe they were her parents. And here is a fundamental difference between a plant and a human. A snapdragon is a snapdragon regardless of where it is planted, regardless of the composition of the soil or lack of soil. It doesn't have to *believe* it's a snapdragon, it doesn't have to be *told* it's a snapdragon, it simply follows the DNA blueprint. As humans, we also follow our DNA blueprint, *and* as we develop, we possess free will and the capacity to imagine and interpret our environments. Anyone who provides basic needs to a young child who has barely if ever had those basic needs met can be *imagined* into "Mom and Dad." This is how Mom came to believe these people were her parents.

Snapdragons prefer well-draining loamy soil. Loamy soil is a mix of sand, silt, and clay. Unless a plant is moved, it will live in one place for the entirety of its life; if the soil is less than optimum, it will not thrive. Clay soil on its own is dense and drains poorly. Root rot will occur if the clay becomes waterlogged. Sand on its own has poor nutrient content and drains water faster than a plant may be able to absorb it. Silt is nutrient rich. Composed of medium-sized particles, it retains nutrients and water at a rate that promotes growth. This couple began to add some sand and silt to the clay that had predominated in Mom's early years.

Chapter Three: Snapdragons

Does a mother feel pain when she gives her child away? I have to believe this might be one of the greatest pains. Thankfully, I have never had to experience it. When snapdragons are pruned early and before they flower, they will grow lateral branches, resulting in stronger stems and more abundant inflorescence. My grandmother must have hoped this desperate move would give Mom a chance to grow stronger, to branch out and create the potential for more blooms.

I'm not sure how long Mom lived with this couple, but I believe it was two or three years. Mom's memories of this time are happy ones. She was being cared for. She was *seen*. She told me they loved her. In Mom's heart and Mom's head, these were her parents.

On a normal day, like any other day, Mom was out running errands with the man she now called father. She had become especially close with him and tagged along whenever she could. When they returned home, a stranger's car sat in the driveway and her mother was talking to a woman *"dressed in fancy clothes"* as Mom would always describe it. She opened the car door and stepped out. Mom would always pause at this point in the story and close her eyes. Her somatic sensations of this event remained intact even decades later.

She knew immediately by the way the adults looked at her that something bad was about to go down. *A familiar feeling began to wash over her. This is what happens when we know persistent trauma. Waiting for the next shoe to drop becomes part of our DNA blueprint—a built-in safety mechanism that alerts us to danger. She could feel that which she could not see. Mom's root system was about to get yanked out.* Maybe this is when Mom's breathing issues really started. She held her breath, she was afraid to breathe. She stood rooted. Her mother walked over and took her by the hand. Mom resisted. "It's OK, come with me," her mother prodded. "She's a nice lady who is just going to take you on a ride for some ice cream." Mom would tell us she didn't want to go on a ride with the nice lady. It was drilled into our heads as children, *"Never get in a car with a stranger. Under any circumstances. No matter what."*

Mom didn't want any ice cream. Mom wanted to stay right where she was. Despite her fear, and with her parents' reassurance, Mom drove away in

Chapter Three: Snapdragons

the front seat of the car with the fancy lady. Mom's small suitcase of personal belongings had already been tucked into the trunk of the car. *The plant had been culled.* What Mom remembers well about this moment is the lady from the Children's Aid Society telling her, "Those are not your parents. You will never see them again. You need to forget them." Turns out Mom had been a placeholder. The couple were now expecting their own child and didn't feel they could afford to keep Mom any longer. She believes she was five or six when this happened. When my own daughter turned five, I tried to imagine what it would be like for her if a stranger suddenly showed up and told her I was not her mother. To be honest, it is not even in my repertoire of emotion to imagine, and for that I am eternally grateful.

Mom was made a permanent ward of the Children's Aid Society. For the next ten years she was moved from foster home to foster home. *She was not thriving.* I think her strong sense of self-preservation dictated most of her decisions during these years. She became desperate to get out from under the control of the Ontario Children's Aid Society. She met my father at a baseball game. He was the pitcher. A young, good-looking Italian bad boy with large deep brown eyes and chiseled features. A star athlete. *A way out.*

Officially, Mom was a ward of the Children's Aid Society until she turned eighteen. She wanted to marry my father, but they were denied permission because of their young age—they were both sixteen. In 1956 there was one way to remedy their dilemma, and that was to get pregnant. So, at the age of barely seventeen my mother became pregnant, was emancipated, and married my father. They moved into my father's childhood home on the farm with Nona and Nonno (my father's parents), my father's brothers, his sister and her husband, and a couple of farm dogs. *"Out of the kettle and into the fire" comes to mind as I write this.*

When I walk into the house to retrieve a vase for the snapdragons, my sister has helped Mom to her chair and made her a cup of tea. Mom is tucked into her chair watching her. She has a soft crooked smile on her face as my sister sings, "I've got the joy, joy, joy, joy down in my heart…" Silent tears are running down my sister's cheeks as the words carry the vibrato of her sorrow. As if to convince herself, she

Chapter Three: Snapdragons

starts dancing a little jig. We *can* show up as joy for Mom. We all feel the complexity of these moments. Compartmentalization isn't working for any of us right now. Especially if we want to stay present. We are learning we can hold much more emotion than we ever imagined. We *can* feel sadness and joy at the same time. Right now, we are treading waters far outside of our usual realm of reality.

Mom calls these snapdragons volunteers because they return every year as if they are a hardy perennial. Some snapdragons are considered tender annuals, and do not overwinter, especially in colder climates like Ontario. These snapdragons have returned all four years in the garden. They pop up randomly and are left to flourish where they bloom. This is how it was for Mom as a child. She had to learn how to flourish where she was planted, even when the conditions were less than ideal. Even when the soil was scarce and lacked nutrients. *Even when she felt like she had been planted in rocks.* Snapdragons are some of the last bloomers to die off. Mom's health has imitated these snapdragons by bouncing back again and again and again when we thought she could not, when we were told she would not.

Cutting the stem, I can't help but pinch off one of the flower heads that has the distinct shape of a pair of dragon lips. I smile as I am transported back to the three- or four-year-old version of myself standing with Mom in her garden. Mom was twenty-one or twenty-two. She is pinching the lips that open the mouth of the *dragon* disguised as a flower in a playful way while she pretends to pinch me on my cheek with the petals. I still can't pass a summer season without picking off a snapdragon flower and repeating this gesture. The lure of opening those lips always outweighs my fear of getting stung, as large bumblebees love to land on snapdragons for pollination.

My grandmother *couldn't* be playful when Mom was a child. There were too many plants and the conditions were harsh. She was in survival mode. I recognize now how much of Mom's mothering has been an attempt to rectify *her* losses. The complication has shown up when my sisters and I are not sure if Mom wants to be the *mother or the child*.

More than once, after hearing a story from Mom's early childhood, I had encouraged her to consider therapy. "Do it, Mom. Get rid of this baggage from the past. Don't carry it any longer. It's a lot. Too much.

Chapter Three: Snapdragons

Don't carry it into your next life." She couldn't. She told me repeatedly, "I can't. I'm tired. I can't relive it all again. It would kill me. I don't want to talk about it." For a long time, Mom relied on the priest for guidance, but ultimately the only person she would completely rely on was herself. Her life had taught her that lesson over and over and over again.

Going through therapy myself, coupled with the healing power of yoga and somatic philosophy and movement, taught me how to show up for Mom in the biggest, brightest way I possibly could for the last three months of her life. When we started talking about MAID, I decided that I would harness all of my life skills and show up unconditionally to the best of my ability. *I didn't need anything from her.*

I place the snapdragons on the table by Mom's chair. She has drifted off to sleep after my sister's serenade. I want these yellow snapdragons with their strength and joy to be the first thing she sees, but when Mom wakes, her fear is palpable and blinds her to the beauty of the flowers. I can feel it before I see it in her weary damp eyes. She is not able to fend off the tears that are rolling down her cheeks. My heart is anxious to ease her suffering and vacillates between surrender to my own fear and a call to action. *But what action?*

There is a constant dialogue taking place between my head and my heart these days over how much Mom wants to talk about MAID. I tentatively ask her if she is crying because she is afraid to die. "Not at all, dear. My heart is aching about leaving behind my children. I love every one of you so much. *I know* how much you will hurt when I am gone, but I have to go. I can't handle this pain anymore. I don't *want* to handle this pain any longer. *I am ready to die.* I feel like such a burden to you and your sisters…"

"No, Mom, you are not a burden. I wish there was more we could do to make it easier. Look at the snapdragons, Mom. I can't believe they are still blooming. Yellow, your favorite color. Do you think if I bring some seeds home, they will germinate?"

We spend the next while squeezing the dry brown seedheads and carefully shaking the minuscule seeds onto a sheet of white paper. Hundreds of tiny black specks hold the potential for new growth. The complex mysteries of life and death are hidden in these tiny seeds that lie dormant now and then somehow transform into the brilliant flowers I see in

Chapter Three: Snapdragons

Mom's vase. Mom is preparing to go dormant. *There is that which we can see and that which we can't see.* In my travel bag I tuck a sealed envelope of the snapdragon seeds that Mom has carefully marked with planting instructions so I can bring Mom's garden home.

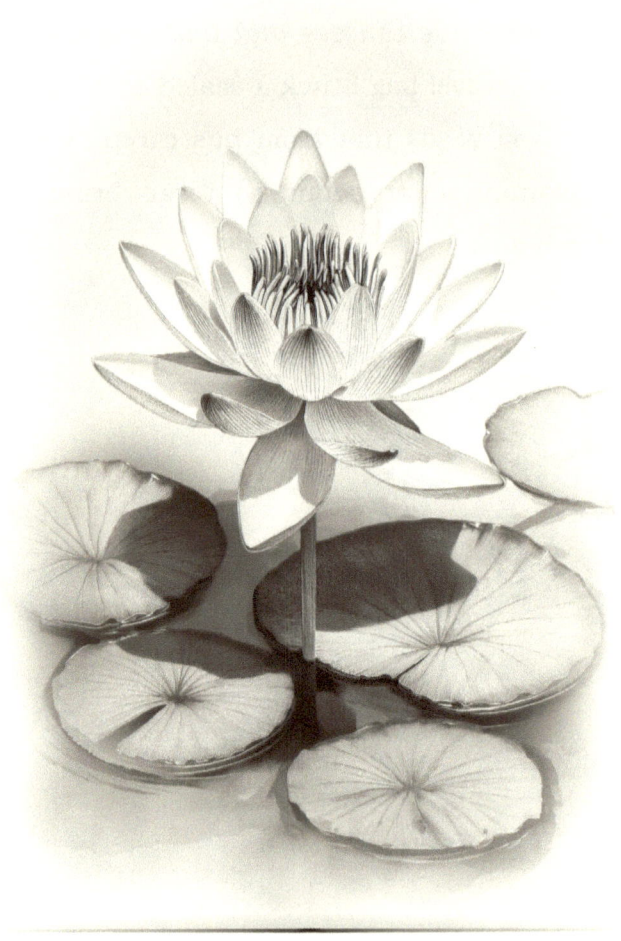

Nymphaeaceae
Common Name – Water Lily
These exquisite star-shaped flowers that float on the surface of the water are a reminder that beauty can surface from an obscure and murky unknown.

Chapter Four

Water Lilies

Journal entry September 16, 2020. The resplendent beauty of nature reflected in Mom's garden is like a compounded salve that has become a healing balm for my tender heart. Verdant leaves have spent their summer drinking in the sun's elixir. In accordance with the season, they are now dropping and have earned a rest from the activity of growing. Mom has earned a rest from the activity of inhabiting her earthly body. Sixty days until November 15.

Fallen leaves will safeguard roots that have spent the summer storing water and nutrients for the cold of winter. Like Mom's pantry in the fall with jars full, the roots will drip-feed their stores to sustain the sleeping plants through their dormancy. In the spring, the stored nutrients will support new growth for the coming season. If I pay attention, it is clear nature is conspiring to guide me through Mom's transition. To show me that transition is really extraordinarily ordinary. *Permanence is the illusion.* There is a divine plan.

The bright sun and warm air have lured Mom into the garden for her morning tea. With a portable oxygen machine and her walker, we choose a comfortable spot at the wrought iron table beside the pond, which is full of activity. Common sparrows flit in and out like locals who navigate their space with familiar ease. We watch them quietly. These shared moments of silence are precious. We can release the effort of grasping for words that seem inadequate and simply feel each other. We process *everything* through our bodies. Neurologically, our first response to any stimulus occurs physically, whether we are aware of it or not, and most of the time we are not. I can feel Mom's gut is roiling this morning. For a time, I stay the course and then I speak, "You don't have to go through with this, Mom. It's OK to change your mind." "I know," she replies softly ... and that is that.

The distant language of cars and church bells give voice to this city where I spent a chunk of my

Chapter Four: Water Lilies

childhood before moving to the farm. It has been forty years since I left, but I still call it *home*. My sisters live here. Their families live here. My mom lives here—*for sixty more days*. My brother Paul lived here. My eyes take in his worn and weary steel-toed work boots. They have had a place of honor in Mom's garden since his premature death. He would love the red geraniums now inhabiting his boots, and I pinch the dried and shriveled petals off the plants. I can't bear to pull up the entire plant because right now that feels like too much loss.

This city looks different than the memory my child-eyes stored. There are still stately old brick and stone houses with fancy slate shingles, leaded glass windows and turrets. Their wrap-around porches boast wooden swings that dangle from chains. The white bead-board cladding that spans their ceilings gives us a hint of the splendor that lies within. Gigantic chestnut and maple trees still line the streets. Intricate dark wrought iron fences still surround these grand homes. That part is the same.

What is different is the ever-increasing number of buildings struggling to maintain their former glory. Single-family homes now hold two or three families in small awkward versions of themselves. Porches are dressed in ill-fitting clothes, and porch swings have been replaced with broken lawn chairs. Once-manicured hedges look long forgotten, and beautiful gardens are overgrown and filled with weeds. The streets are now home for far too many who have become strangers in their own town. Socio-economic hardship, mental health issues, and drug and alcohol abuse are not so hidden on many of these city blocks. Mom's street is a little of both versions.

My brother knew these streets. He had been surrendered to the Children's Aid Society at age thirteen as a last resort. His needs seemed to have exceeded what my parents could offer. There was a real concern that his escapades had just been practice for something bigger that would take not only Paul, but my parents down with him. The judge had advised my parents to make this drastic decision. Mom was trying to outrun her story, but we only know what we know and we don't know what we don't know. I believe Mom felt guilty about this her entire life. She knew what it was like to be tethered to the foster care system.

Chapter Four: Water Lilies

My brother was a scavenger and a hoarder who long ago sold most of Mom's nice jewelry and anything else of value to support his drug and alcohol habit. He had a huge heart and always planned to pay her back tenfold, but he was never able to break up with the substances that kept him in a chemical prison.

The day he died, it was Mom who found him in his apartment. We had waited years to get him into rent-controlled housing that provided some services and monitored the residents. By this time, he was on disability. The police in town had known him for years. In order to satisfy his addiction, he had resorted to behaviors that led to stints in jail and prison for aggravated assaults and theft. He wanted to die. He told me so. Often. His life had been reduced to doing anything it took to avoid going through withdrawal. He was depleted. *He had used all of the stored energy in his roots.* Four years later, Mom still sleeps with a piece of sleeve from his flannel shirt tucked close to her heart. She prays the Rosary for him every night.

Perennials can live for several years, and some can live for decades. *Integration and disintegration.*

When my sister called to let me know Paul had died, silent tears rolled down my cheeks while a sense of relief softened my sadness. He had been dying on a painful installment plan for most of his life. Now he was free. Mom was free. We were free. I know Mom is counting on seeing him again. I won't miss this house or this block or this city, but today I feel grateful for this home and this garden and the neighbors who have stepped up to help Mom when she needed it.

An antique hand pump has been retrofitted to deliver the steady stream of water circulating in the pond. I know this hand pump from our farm. Spats over whose turn it was to go outside in the cold and pump the next bucket reverberated through the house when we were young. We relied on this pump to draw up the cold spring-fed drinking water from the old shallow well by the side door. By now, we were living in the country on a twenty-acre farm. City water was not an option. My parents had been flipping houses before flipping houses was a thing. We had moved six times before I reached the seventh grade and we settled on the farm. This was their dream home. A place where my father could breed

Chapter Four: Water Lilies

and train standardbred horses, and my mother could grow a garden and raise her four children.

Mom's organic vegetable garden was prolific, feeding six of us for much of the year. Most plants are autotrophic and have the ability to manufacture their own food using light, water, carbon dioxide, and other chemicals. Autotrophs are considered *producers* because of their ability to manufacture their own food. Humans are heterotrophic—*consumers* who rely on producers or outside sources to nourish us. In summer we ate fresh vegetables straight from the garden. Farm to table wasn't an expensive elite fad, but a way of feeding your family. Food was bountiful, and there was always room for one more at the kitchen table.

In autumn, Mason jars full of the season's colorful harvest would fill the old wooden shelves in the musty damp dugout basement. The old basement stairs were so creaky, it was like navigating land mines whenever we kids attempted to sneak some Christmas bakery or other goodies from their hiding places in the pantry. Mom learned how to grow food, how to preserve food, and how to prepare food as a tangible expression of her love *and* a guarantee that she would not go hungry again. She was happiest when she was cooking for her family.

Mom no longer has the stamina to stand in the kitchen and cook food. After an exhaustive search in the local area, she has found a service that delivers prepared meals. I deduce her main criteria for choosing this particular service is the *desserts*. Mom has a sweet tooth that has benefited all of us over the years. It was our ritual to go to the local grocer on Friday nights, and whoever accompanied Mom was guaranteed some excessive sugary sweet treat on the way home. No dinner was served without dessert. While these prepared meals provide Mom with adequate nutrition, they lack curiosity and creativity. *They look tired on arrival.* All the cakes Mom has baked over the years surface in my memory as I hand her a piece of ho-hum-looking carrot cake. "Here you go, Mom. Why don't you eat dessert first." I miss Mom's cooking. Even though her appetite is small and sporadic these days, she insists on keeping her cupboards full. Years of going hungry as a child will not allow for any empty space in her pantry.

As I dig up the gladiolus bulbs in one section of the garden, an orchestra of birds accompanies the

Chapter Four: Water Lilies

oxygen tank whirring a steady beat. Mom is cleaning the corms after I dig them up. These swollen, underground containers wrapped in dried leaves store the nutrients and starch the plants will need to survive the winter and resume active growth in the spring. Next spring will be different as my sisters and I will not be pooling our funds to acquire Mom's annual gift certificate to the local nursery.

With her eyes closed, Mom's face is turned toward the sun as if she is a heliotropic plant who opens and closes her petals daily according to when she can absorb the most sunlight. Heliotropic plants literally follow the path of the sun throughout the day in an effort to feed themselves. Phototropism is the movement of plants toward or away from *any* light source. The morning glories, moonflowers, daisies, daylilies, and poppies in Mom's garden all exhibit some form of tropism.

Mom's days are becoming shorter as she spends more and more time in bed away from the light and folded up for rest. I watch her sensorily draw the sunlight inward and I pause to join her. Every second counts these days. The moments arrive like a double-edged sword: one edge carving time into precious moments for new memories to be made, while the other edge cuts off chunks of time that can never be recovered. I can't think of that right now or I will miss these last days with Mom by forfeiting them to an imaginary future that will have stolen our priceless time.

The pond is filled with large green lily pads vying for space on the crowded surface of the water. Plants that live in soil grow extensive and elaborate root systems to search out and store water. Not so for water lilies. They *live* in water unencumbered by the burden of having to search out and collect this precious compound made when two hydrogen atoms and one oxygen atom bind. These round waxy lily pads and their water lilies appear to hover on the gently rippling surface of the water, but they are actually connected to the bottom of the pond by a fine floating stem and root system.

So it is with Mom and her three daughters. We are impersonating lily pads right now as we *appear* to be free-floating on the top of the water, with each of us vying for our place in a pond that sometimes feels too dark and too deep with too many unknowns. When one of us slips below the surface, the others manage to stay afloat. We are tethered together by an invisible cord made from bits of matter that have landed us in this place at this time.

Nymphaeaceae is the scientific name for the water lily family. These exquisite star-shaped flowers that float on the surface of the water are a reminder that beauty *can* surface from an obscure and murky unknown. *There is that which we can see and that which we cannot see...* All of life—including death—uses contrast to teach us what we value.

When my sisters and I became parents, our priorities shifted to nurturing and protecting *our* seedlings. Over many years, we individually and collectively did our best to step out of the family drama that had defined our early lives. We made purposeful choices that would nurture and increase the vitality of our family units. Like phototropic plants, we were turning toward the light.

Most water lilies close at night and open in the morning. Petioles connect the center of a peltate or round waxy leaf blade to the soil on the floor of the pond. Each water lily has one shoot that rises vertically from modified stems called rhizomes. These shoots can grow over six feet long to reach the water's surface. Rhizomes are secret containers that live below the earth's surface, where they store nutrients for the plant. They anchor the plant, deliver oxygen to the roots, and form new shoots in the spring after a plant has died back in the winter. They allow plants to survive harsh seasons underground.

If a rhizome is cut in half, each half is capable of producing a new node or shoot from which a flower will grow, although it may require some extra time. As humans, we bring our lived experiences to every given moment. Stored not in rhizomes but in the containers of our bodies, minds, and hearts, these experiences invisibly feed us the nutrients we need to sustain us now and in the future. My sisters and I are growing our ability to rise up like these water lily shoots each time we choose to stay present for Mom and for each other. I trust that if this experience metaphorically cuts us in half, with time we will grow a new shoot.

Water lilies crave the sun and prefer to inhale six hours of the full bright sunlight that will be converted from light energy to chemical energy. Think Krebs cycle. Stomata are microscopic pores covering the surface of the leaves so they can take in carbon dioxide and release oxygen. All plants have stomata. Lily pads are unique by virtue of the placement of their stomata only on the top of the leaf that is not submerged in water. Their round dish-like shape and waxy top coating helps keep the stomata open, so the process of respiration can flow for this unique aquatic plant.

We do this in reverse with every breath we take. Delivering oxygen to our cells with each inhalation and expelling carbon dioxide with each exhalation. In Mom's case, her lungs no longer have enough surface area to exchange these gases efficiently or effectively. Lily pads use the surface area of their waxy leaves to maximize the process of respiration. We use the surface area of our lungs, which are filled with millions of *alveoli* that resemble minuscule clusters of grapes. A healthy lung has a surface area that could cover a tennis court if spread out. When chronic obstructive pulmonary disease (COPD) sets in, the alveoli begin to rupture in response to inhaled irritants. These ruptured areas form pockets called *blebs,* greatly reducing the surface area available for gas exchange. Mom's supplemental oxygen helps but is no substitute for her own physiology.

When Mom was first prescribed oxygen, she would take it off whenever she could. Now she is dependent on this mechanical version of a lung and becomes anxious without it.

I have completed digging up the gladiolus bulbs, and Mom is helping me clean and sort them. Anything that is soft to the touch or dried out goes into the compost. The rest are spread out on newspaper where they will dry in the sun. Once they're dried, their winter habitat will become a recycled onion bag that hangs in my sister's basement for the winter. We are all thrilled to have any small piece of Mom's garden to bring home to our own gardens. We believe we can keep a bit of Mom close through her flowers.

A single water lily still blooms. The sun is reflecting off the abundant petals that display the shades of purple spiraling toward the center. Some varieties of water lilies have up to two hundred petals that merge into one exquisite corolla. I consider water lilies to be part magic. In Alice's Wonderland these petals might form a delicate purple teacup resting on a green lily pad saucer. Mom asks me to go inside and fetch her iPad. She wants more information on

Chapter Four: Water Lilies

water lilies. I have learned to seek knowledge by watching my mother with her fifth-grade education continuously seek knowledge.

As children in the sixties, we had the full set of Encyclopedia Britannica. The imposing gold-embossed edges mimicking the Bible demanded a certain level of respect. This was a huge investment for my parents, and they were proud to have afforded these important learning tools for us. I am mindful to voice each of these memories to Mom as they surface. I want her to leave knowing every good thing she has ever given me over the span of my life. The time for old grievances has passed for me. We have both done our best. "You know what I admire about you, Mom? Your curiosity and your fearlessness. Ever since I can remember, you have been a seeker of practical knowledge. Thank you for modeling that for me."

We discover water lilies are dichogamous, meaning the pistils and stamens mature at different times to prevent self-pollination. The pistils or female sex organs mature on the first day the plant blooms. The stamens or male sex organs follow and crowd together in the center, forming a deep orange-yellow circle with their tips dipped in purple. We learn rhizomes are edible! Water lily rhizomes can be eaten broiled, boiled, baked, raw, or dried and ground into flour. I look at Mom and she looks at me. "Not today, Mom. We already have dinner planned." The rhizomes have gained a reprieve.

We decide to leave the pond running for now. Mom enjoys hearing the water dance between the pump and the pond's surface while watching the birds splash in the water. It takes us twice as long to get inside the house as it did to come out. Mom heads straight for her bed and I cover her with a warm blanket, kiss her forehead, and turn out the light.

Part Two

AUTUMN'S GIFTS

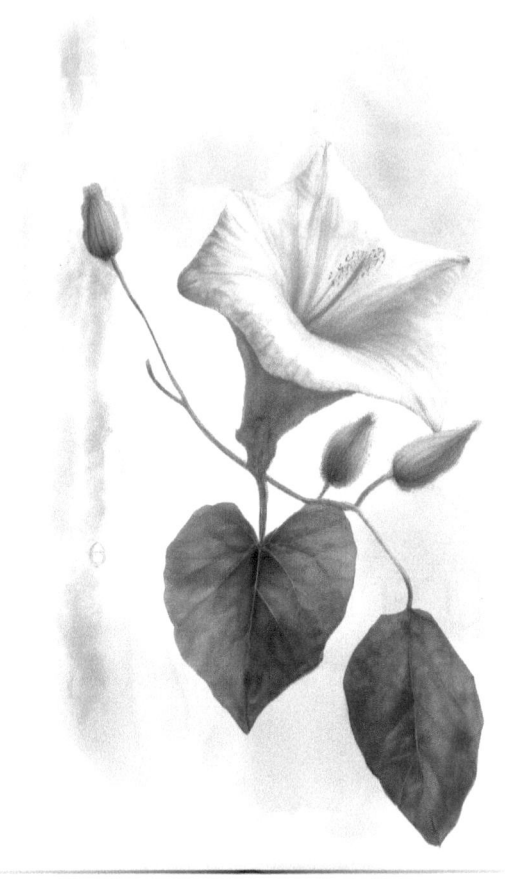

Ipomoea alba
Common Name – Moonflower

Moonflowers symbolize transformation. When the flower head opens, we see it is possible to reflect light out of the darkness. This process describes the theme for our time together right now. Mom is still alive!

Chapter Five

MOONFLOWER

Languidly taking over one corner of the garden, a large sprawling vine spills under, over, and between the pickets. Meandering onto the city sidewalk, it occasionally grazes an unsuspecting ankle. Uneven cracks have recorded the history of the seasons in the sidewalks of this city block. This is Ontario. While the seasons have become blurred with changing weather patterns, they are still distinct. Nature lives and dies by rhythmical, cyclical, seasonal elements. Heart-shaped forest-green leaves six inches wide and six inches long contrast with the gray concrete. They look robust next to neighboring plants whose leaves are now tinged in browns and curling at the edges. Others have floated to the ground at the seasonal urging of their DNA.

The leaves belong to a plant Mom calls moonflower. I let the vein structure of this leaf mandala mesmerize me. A respite from the circular thinking that wants to run my brain these days. A chance for my nervous system to regulate my breath and check in with my heart. The petiole is where the leaf and stem connect. Extending vertically from the base up the center of each leaf to the apex or tip is a first-order vein. This is the largest and strongest vein in the leaf and moves water and nutrients from the stem into the leaves. Branching off the first-order vein are secondary and tertiary veins that ensure distribution into the furthest reaches of each leaf.

I study the veins on the back of my own hand. According to the Cleveland Clinic, our vascular system has sixty thousand miles of veins, arteries, and capillaries. Unlike plants, which rely on pressure gradients to move water and nutrients, we rely on a pump. The pumping action of the heart moves oxygen-rich arterial blood from the left side of the heart to muscles, tissues, and organs, where capillaries exchange oxygen for carbon dioxide. Oxygen-poor venous blood then returns to the right side of the heart through the veins and into the lungs, where carbon dioxide is exchanged for oxygen, and the cycle repeats itself.

Chapter Five: Moonflower

For plants, transpiration or evaporation of water from the surface of the leaves via stomata creates a pressure gradient that continuously draws the water upward from the roots to the leaves. The pressure in Mom's vascular system has been high for many years now. I equate Mom's high blood pressure with the beginning of her end. I wonder if plants experience their own version of high blood pressure.

I remember Mom's legs covered in large lumpy reddish-blue veins that traveled crooked paths and looked like a relief map. To my child's eyes, they did not belong on the legs of my beautiful young mother. Superficial varicose veins can develop as a result of pregnancy. In her late twenties at this time, she was already a mother to four living children and two deceased. Surgeries to remove these angry veins would give her some respite from the pain, but even more insidious was the process taking place *inside* her arteries.

There is that which we can see and that which we cannot see. Plaque was slowly, quietly, and perniciously building up and reducing the blood flow in the major arteries that fed her heart and the rest of her vital organs. Not only does this process inhibit free blood flow throughout the system, but it can also make the flow turbulent. *Turbulent blood flow tends to clot.* Clots in the heart's arteries (*coronary arteries*) cause heart attacks. A clot in the carotid arteries in our neck can break free, float up to our brain, and cause a stroke. It is a testament to the tenacity of our physiology that this disease is often silent until our arteries are 80 to 90% occluded.

Mom calls the moonflower "an exotic plant." She pauses and takes a deliberate breath supported by tiny plastic prongs that deliver oxygen through her nose. "I've never grown one before." I love that Mom is still curious, even with death close. Moonflowers are large white exotic members of the *Convolvulaceae* family, whose familiar name is *morning glory*. Like all members of the morning glory family, they love to wrap and wind their way up any vertical structure. Mom envisioned this moonflower might wrap itself around the wrought iron scrolls of railing leading up to her front door. Thigmotropism is a plant's response to touch or contact with things in its environment. Think sweet peas. I imagine myself morphing into a thigmotropic plant and wrapping myself around

Chapter Five: Moonflower

my mother's limbs and torso as I gradually wind myself inside to gently encircle her heart.

Folklore has it that moonflowers are mystical and magical because they only bloom at night, and magical things occur in the dark of the night. The corollas are one to two inches wide and reminiscent of the flowers on trumpet vines. Creamy white petals tinted with violet centers contrast with the forest-green leaves. Right now, these petals are relaxed and more closed than open. In the evening, they will unfurl into large round milky corollas the size of small dinner plates. Thought to symbolize *transformation*, when the flower head opens, we see it is possible to reflect light out of the darkness. This process describes the theme for our time together right now. *Mom is still alive!* We are choosing to focus on life rather than death. We are choosing to view death as *transformation* rather than the end.

As it has for humans, the biology of plants has evolved and adapted to changing environments in order to maximize chances for survival. One bonus can be even more stunning displays of color, texture, scent, and innovation. Many of these plants have been modified at the hands of man to better suit his needs. For the plant, the single driving force is survival. Humans have this driving force too. I have spent a good deal of time pondering our *will to live*. We want to live longer and we want brighter and better versions of ourselves. We want it to be easy. Many of us struggle to invest the *time* and *energy* it takes to create these bright, light versions of ourselves, too distracted and busy by a culture driven to be successful on the *outside*.

We modify humans with medicine and surgery and machines. *Mom has been modified.* Her internal environment no longer supports vitality. Moonflowers rely on nocturnal pollinators like bats and moths in place of the butterflies and bees that pollinate flowers by day. My lack of experience cannot determine whether these moonflowers are doing the *plant version of sleep* or are ready to be deadheaded. When I ask Mom, she smiles. "Those aren't dead, dear. We'll come back tonight when the moon is out and the sky is dark, and you'll see."

Journal entry September 26, 2020. Mom is still full of bits and pieces of information she wants to pass on to us before she leaves. We are experiencing some lovely warm late September

Chapter Five: Moonflower

days. Tonight, I could tell Mom was tired and ready for bed, but she insists on waiting for the night sky to show me the beauty of her moonflowers. There are so many mother-seeds she wants to plant before she leaves her body, and communication between us becomes an ethereal sensing we will learn to trust over time. I know her sense of urgency because I feel it also.

I have resisted the urge to coddle her. Some days I think how auspicious it would be if she stepped into the garden and keeled over. That would be OK—even better than MAID. I have already formulated a plan ... no CPR, call my sisters, hold her... but what if she's not all the way dead? My secret wish is that she will die on her own before her birthday. If that's in her garden, all the better. Fifty-one days until November 15.

Caressing my skin, the warmth of the night air soothes me. The sky is clear and illuminated with white light that pours off the surface of the moon. The moon is in a *waxing gibbous phase*. It is sixty-seven percent illuminated. A moon is *waxing* when it is fifty to one-hundred percent illuminated. *Gibbous* describes the oval to round shape we observe in the night sky. In fact, the moon's light is *actually* a reflection of the sun's light bouncing off a dark gray round rock that has no light source of its own. An illusion we have embraced in script and song. *There is that which we can see and that which we cannot see...*

Mom taught us to sing "By the Light of the Silvery Moon" when we were young. She worked at Valleyview Nursing Home as a nurse's aide. One or two residents often graced our dinner table on a Sunday evening. We learned these songs so we could sing them for the elderly residents who lived at Valleyview. Something saved in the recesses of their memories would awaken as they sang along with us. A respite from tedious hours spent waiting to die.

My sisters and I have laughed at Mom's fierce determination to turn us into the next incarnation of the Andrews Sisters. We were part of Mom's fairytale family. The family she conjured up from books and radio and television. *The family she thought everyone had but her.* We are five days away from the full moon. Taking in the splendor of this giant reflective orb, I am embraced by a delicate sweet scent. Closing my eyes, I draw the scent inward with a long slow deep inhalation. I feel the air entering and filling my nostrils, touching the back of my throat, and moving

Chapter Five: Moonflower

into my heart center... I feel it touch all my cells. It borders on intoxication. *I am being charged like a crystal by the energy of the moon.*

"Look, Theresa," Mom half whispers, and I see the tulip flowers open into huge white replicas of the full moon right before our eyes. Now I know *why* this plant has the name moonflower. They have six-inch-deep inner cavities connecting the petals to the stem. These nocturnal plants only bloom at night. It is dark except for the moon and stars illuminating the large round white flowers. When I look at Mom, her eyes appear translucent. She gazes back at me, and we hold our gaze to draw each other in. The vastness of the universe is reflected in our eyes, as we silently acknowledge that there is so much more than our humanness can comprehend. Mom is ready for bed. When I tuck her in, I am silently giving thanks that she is still here.

> *Journal entry September 27, 2020 (Sunday). My sisters and I took a magical, mystical ride with Mom and the help of some psilocybin mushrooms. She was all in. We have been listening to a lot of Alan Watts and other philosophers and pondering their thoughts on death and dying. Our intent in*

taking the mushrooms was to connect beyond the boundaries of our everyday minds and hearts and bodies that are preoccupied with the mundane so we might step into the mystical. A moment to further grow a safe place for all of us to show up for each other. Forty-nine days until November 15.

As if preparing for a sacred ceremony, we ready the private space in my sister's enchanting back yard. Surrounded by mature gardens, forty-year-old trumpet vines, ancient maples, and the sounds of chickadees and their chickadee-dee-dee-dee calls, nature wraps us in her arms. The sun is bright and I thank the universal God for giving us this glorious day to explore. A blazing red maple tree grows beside the deck. Its iridescent red-orange colors are transforming the green leaves into a fiery showcase against the dark textural bark.

As she sits on a comfy lawn chair, we tuck Mom into a soft blanket version of a womb. We burn sage to cleanse the space and prepare each of us so we might show up without fear for the plant medicine. My brother-in-law has brewed the mushrooms into a tea. He is serving the tea in miniature ceramic Japanese teacups, and he promises to be close in case we need anything. A soda biscuit and peanut butter will wash down the strong, pungent taste of the mushrooms. With "Speak to Me" by Pink Floyd playing in the background, we toast to a beneficial journey and drink the tea....

We sob from the depths of our souls. We laugh from the depths of our souls. We *feel* the contract we have made with each other and as a family. We create a safe space for all of it. Mom describes kaleidoscopes of colors and shapes as people are passing by and looking at her with love. Seeing loved ones who have already journeyed out of their bodies is a common phenomenon reported by many as they move closer to death. Mom feels like she is being welcomed home. The woman we knew as Grandma has appeared. The one foster mother who really cared for Mom for the two or three years she was with that family. She would have been eleven-ish years old.

She sees her birth mother and feels only love. She feels the love from her family that she has craved all of her life. In this moment she understands that they have done their best. She sees me as a strong warrior and tells me to never forget that I carry this in me. "You can do anything, Theresa. You are a warrior. You are meant to do great things. The world needs you." When "My Sweet Lord" by George Harrison starts playing in the background, Mom knows this is the song she wants to hear as she takes flight from her body. We make a pact. *George Harrison is now part of this journey.*

While I'm resting my palms on Mom's feet, a bright white light that I know will welcome and enfold her fills my vision. I sense it would welcome *me* right now, but it is not yet my time. I tell her, "Don't be afraid, Mom. I am witnessing the light, and it is a glorious and welcoming light that is filled with *only* love." Next, a gut-wrenching sensation squeezes my entire being, and I know I have begun separating from Mom already. I feel the light and the dark. I am *eviscerated* by my sorrow. A guttural sob bursts forth from me, and then ... I begin to dance.

I dance away anything in me that might prevent me from letting go of Mom completely. I dance away the *angst* that interferes with my love for my sisters. I dance away the *void* that fills the space where things that are no longer useful once resided. When my deep sobs are complete, I am compelled to continue dancing. I can feel myself filling with joy and love and freedom. I am a whirling dervish moving to the rhythm of the universe. When I stop dancing, it is not by choice, but by the same timing that underlies all of nature. I lay my spent body, mind, heart, and soul under the blazing red maple. I am enveloped in complete and utter silence. I am done. I am ready. I can do this. *I was made for this moment.*

This time is tender, joyful, and sad. Mom grows quieter every day. Her eyes are becoming increasingly distant, yet they still shine. I begin to suspect that Mom is already hovering between two worlds. This second world remains a mystery to those of us who can only remember the experience of our present life, but I feel Mom has touched this place and holds the secret like a moonflower waiting for dusk. I believe I touched this place with the help of the plant medicine. The bright white light I saw during our ceremony on Sunday looks just like the full moon I am taking in now.

The large white moonflowers back home in Mom's garden are mimicking the moon. I wonder, will Mom sail past the moon on the way out of her body? Will she touch the moon? *Is she already a part of the moon?* I look at Mom's eyes and I see the *fullness* of Mom the human being, the *essence* of Mom the spirit in human form, the *wisdom* of 80 years lived, the *mischievous* Mom, the *tired* Mom, the Mom who loves us. *I see her love.* If you leave the faded moonflowers, they will form dry brown seedpods. Mom has promised to help me harvest some seeds when they are ready.

Chapter Five: Moonflower

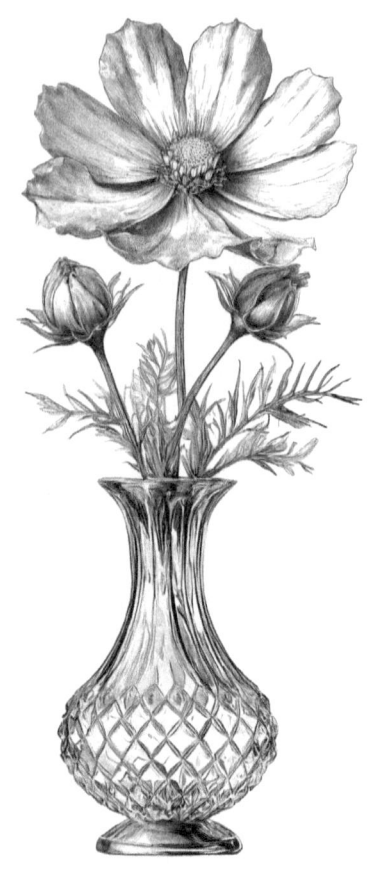

Cosmos bipinnatus
Common Name – Cosmos

Cosmos leaves are the color of healthy spring grass and have a very distinct lacelike quality. They bring a unique texture to the garden, the way we each bring a unique texture to this time with Mom and with each other.

Chapter Six

COSMOS

Journal entry October 12, 2020. *Well, so much for a daily journal. Mom is resting, and I must continue to document these days. On days where I read some of my journal entries, I am already searching for the memory that matches the words I have written. The days go by too fast when I am imagining Mom gone and too slow when I am watching Mom suffer and struggle for her breath. Thirty-four more days if Mom leaves on November 15 as planned.*

The cosmos flowers are still blooming in Mom's garden as if it is mid-summer. I wonder if they feel confused by these exceptionally warm and sunny mid-October days. The Greek origin word for the cosmos flower is *kosmos*. It means *orderly* and *universal order* and refers to the symmetry of the delicate petals. The primary impetus for a plant to begin pouring energy into preparing for dormancy and the quiet of winter is decreasing daylight hours. The cosmos will bloom until the first frost, which is usually mid-October in this area of southwestern Ontario. They have reseeded themselves and are plentiful. The way they appear randomly throughout the garden tells me that the winds have had a hand in where they land. I love how Mom's garden is an equal mix of order and chaos.

I relish every minute with Mom, but it is a lot of sensation to carry in my heart, and I know my sisters feel the same way. The past few days have been filled with an ease that belies the gravity of why we are together. This is the rhythm of life that is always moving us. Sometimes consciously and other times unconsciously. At times we pirouette and at times we trip and fall. If we peel off our layers all the way down to the most elemental version of ourselves, we are all spinning molecules of energy bouncing off of each other. Buried by our compulsion to participate in our human lives, we can forget we are dancing and think the present moment is fixed.

Today's gorgeous sunny skies will require only a light jacket. Mom and I have spent the morning fin-

Chapter Six: Cosmos

ishing gifts for my sister's sixtieth birthday. When we were very young, we could coax Mom into stopping her chores and drawing us paper dolls on used pieces of cardboard saved for just this purpose. These dolls commandeered our imaginations, and we would spend long hours drawing, coloring, and cutting out their wardrobes. No one bought Mom toys. As a child, she learned to make her own toys, and my sisters and I reaped the benefits.

Earthy autumn scents waft into the living room through open windows. Mom's hands and fingers dance slowly with each other as they restring a necklace. These are the hands of an artist. Together, we work in silence. I am sorting through the dried remnants of fall from Mom's garden as I embellish a grapevine wreath for my middle sister. From her lift chair, Mom is gazing upon her garden through eight small panes of glass.

This chair Mom is in right now takes up a lot of the space she once filled with her own unique decorating style. Mom could have been an interior designer, and she passed her passion for aesthetics on to all of us. She was never afraid to learn something new and try out the latest trends. Before they bought the farm, my parents were raising four of us on my father's income from Ford, and money was always tight, but Mom had learned to manifest for herself at a very early age.

When she was still a young girl, she taught herself to sew and earned money stitching Barbie clothes for the girls at school. She taught us how to strip paint off woodwork and how to put paint on walls. She taught us how to remove old wallpaper and how to apply new wallpaper. She taught me to be brave. To occupy my space and make it mine. "It's only paint, Theresa. We can change it if it's not what we like."

Unfortunately, she cannot change this large ugly gray-brown chair. *She hates it.* Just like hospital walls, it seems there is only one color for these chairs, and that is the color that reminds me my mom is not the same. The chair has pockets sewn into the sides that proclaim ease and convenience but are really disguises to hide the fact that Mom can't walk like she once did. Getting out of her chair now requires some assistance. Just as foreign is the rolling side table my husband has modified to hold everything Mom needs within easy reach: her medications, an inhaler, a box of Kleenex, some form of hard candy, the remotes, and two small Mason jars filled with the water she uses when she paints with watercolors.

When I glance at Mom, she is already looking at me. Our eyes take on the sheen of morning dew as they glaze with tears. I move so I can sit on the floor at her feet and rest my head on her lap. We hold each other in a long embrace filled with messages that convey more than words. Ten million sensory nerves carry sensations to our awareness and tell us how raw we are. We are all titrating our emotions right now. Some days we can hold more and other days, less. It is astounding how much we are capable of feeling when we sense we are safe enough to show up vulnerable and open and the other person responds in kind. It's a rare moment as it takes a willingness on the part of both individuals to let down that which guards us and to trust. I am grateful to be mutually wrapped in love with Mom right now.

With our projects finished, Mom has suggested we might take a drive to Grand Bend and the surrounding towns. She wants to take in the shores of Lake Huron one last time. She wants to see this place that has fed her soul for much of her adult life. The physical location that has soothed her when she needed space for healing and shelter from life. Growing up, our family spent countless summer days playing on these shores. When we married and had children, this was the gathering place for our families every summer. Now, our children's children play on these same white sand beaches.

We decide to go on a fossil hunt. Mom has been picking up rocks ever since I can remember, and she taught us to pick up rocks too. This area is rich with brachiopods, horn coral, crinoids, and other stone relics from the very distant past. Brachiopods were alive 545 million years ago—a number my brain struggles to fathom. These fossils are solid, dense, enduring reminders of the infinite cycles of life and death or *integration and disintegration* that are always in motion. It is easy to miss these fossils if you are not focused on looking for them. *There is that which we can see and that which we cannot see.*

Wherever we are and whatever story we are living, we are always in transition. Our cells die and renew with regularity. Some people say that every seven to ten years *all* of our cells have regenerated. Science supports this truth for *most* of our cells, but not *all* of them. Despite this regeneration, we see the reality of aging all around us. Maybe we feel it ourselves when we notice a little more effort is called for in our daily activities. These are the thoughts taking up space in my brain these days. We rarely pay attention to death unless we are being touched by it directly. *Right now, I am being shoved.*

With the aid of a kind stranger, we help Mom walk down to the beach, and I say a silent prayer that there will be another gracious soul when it is time to get her back into the car. Scooping rocks and sand into a bucket, I bring the shore to Mom, who is too unsteady to walk to the water's edge. I have a love-hate relationship with technology, but today I am grateful for the ability to Facetime with my daughter Stephanie. As we show her our treasures, our hearts store one more memory to sustain us through the winter months.

By late afternoon we are both hungry. Mom has been craving English-style fish and chips, so we set off to find a local chip stand. A few bites are all Mom can eat, but each bite stirs a memory stored deep in her taste buds. Most practicing Catholics abstain from meat of any kind and eat only fish on Fridays.

Mom's taste buds awaken a memory of the fresh perch from Lake Erie and the thick, crisp, golden french fries drenched in malt vinegar that were our Friday dinner staple.

She remembers four young children clambering around the table while my father unwrapped the oil-stained newspaper tied with white twine. She remembers how the newspaper served as the plates. How she would slide an equal portion of the fish and chips in front of each of her children. She remembers, and she loves *every. single. bite.*

Mom is not eating much these days. The blood supply that should be feeding her gut for digestion is now reserved for more important organs like the brain. I know how this goes. For years I have harped at Mom about her eating habits: salting every morsel before she tastes it, slathering butter on everything you can slather butter on and some things you just shouldn't, eating too much cheese, too much ice cream, too many sweets. These days I tell her to eat whatever she wants, whenever she wants. To this day, Mom's go-to snack is a saltine soda biscuit loaded with butter. A holdover from her days in the orphanage.

Chapter Six: Cosmos

It's early evening when we turn around to drive 116 kilometers back to Mom's house. It's been a full day. A wonderful day. An epic memory-making day that I will be sure to journal about. Our eyes capture the beauty of blaze oranges, reds, and yellows spanning the horizon as we drive in silence and watch the sun go down. There could be no more acceptable ending to this day than for nature to put on this dazzling display of color. Mom closes her eyes in the passenger seat and I let my thoughts put words to my feelings.

I have the advantage of not living here full-time and therefore not having a family and job and life to keep up during these last days with Mom. I have left all of that behind with an open ticket home and very few distractions. My husband encouraged me to go and stay as long as I needed. I am thankful to be here so completely. So much of our lives have been spent far apart, and it's a precious gift that we have this time together now. The angst of my youth had been falling away for years; at times without me knowing it and other times at the end of a fiery exchange and deliberate reflection.

Mom and I are not the same people we were when she unceremoniously threw me out of the house at the age of fourteen. That day I stuffed my clothes into a green plastic garbage bag, called a friend, and vowed never to ask my parents for another thing as long as I lived. I had my mother's street savvy. I didn't need them. I had imprinted my mother's story over the years and somehow thought this was normal. Lots of kids leave home at fourteen. That was 1973. I didn't return, and my relationship with my parents remained tenuous for several years.

It was my daughter who brought us back together. She was born in June of 1979. By then I was nineteen, living in another country and married to an American. Little by little our mutual love for this innocent baby girl overflowed its container and usurped our hurts.

As my mother dozes beside me and I drive in the deepening dusk, I recall our conversation from a few nights ago. We lay tucked into bed together, and she apologized to me for what happened when I was fourteen.

"How I could have thought that was okay, I will never understand. I broke all my dishes that day."

"I remember, Mom."

"It was what I knew. It was how I was raised. I did my best, but it doesn't feel like it was good enough."

Chapter Six: Cosmos

"I know, Mom."

"I'm sorry, dear."

"Thank you, Mom."

By the time we arrive home from the lake, Mom is exhausted. I struggle to help her up four stairs and into her bedroom. Too weak to lift her leg onto the step, I offer my shoulder as a human cane. We both go down and grapple with each other and the oxygen tube as we crawl up the steps. I listen to the portable machine fall back down the steps. *Thump. thump. thump.* Mom half walks, half stumbles, and collapses onto her bed. I temporarily increase the oxygen to ease the load of breathing and give her a boost. I can't increase it too much as the chemoreceptors in Mom's system have adjusted to higher-than-normal blood levels of carbon dioxide. For those of us without COPD, higher levels of carbon dioxide stimulate us to breathe deeper and with more frequency. Mom's main drive to breathe is no longer carbon dioxide. Instead, now it is low blood oxygen levels. If I give her too much oxygen, I'll diminish that drive and she could stop breathing. I make a mental note to ask the nurse what too much oxygen looks like in Mom's case.

It's a good long while before Mom recovers her breath. I watch her skin regain a modicum of color, although these days it is always pale with shades of grays and blues. My sisters and I have learned to coach Mom in how to slow her breathing and extend her exhalations. Something I learned as a nurse. We breathe along with her when she doesn't have the capacity to digest words. "Do what I am doing, Mom. Let's breathe together." I wonder how families with no medical knowledge do it. How they care for someone with complex medical issues, often on their own. Maybe it's easier not to know.

The *tripod* position is taught to people with COPD. Mom will sit in her chair or on the side of her bed with her legs apart and her elbows resting on the table. Leaning her head on her clasped hands lets her surrender the weight and the effort. Heads are surprisingly heavy and average eleven pounds. This is the weight of a bowling ball. These periods of air hunger are intimidating and evoke feelings of helplessness for all of us—*even me.*

My husband, Pete, lived through colon cancer fifteen years ago. One evening when he was having a severe reaction to his first chemotherapy session,

Chapter Six: Cosmos

I placed a frantic call to the oncologist. I apologized profusely for bothering him. "I should know what to do, I am a nurse." He calmly reassured me, "Right now, you are a wife who is watching her husband struggle. Do not apologize." I will be eternally grateful for his words and permission to be a frightened wife who was watching her husband suffer. I learned that caring for a beloved family member can render the professional me somewhat useless at times.

These are the moments that remind me *why* we are doing the MAID program. I have spent a large part of my life teaching in one capacity or another. A fundamental learning principle is the importance of understanding the *"why."* Without this understanding, it is difficult to move forward for anything with real conviction. On days when Mom is energetic and laughing, second thoughts creep into my head. I never voice these thoughts to Mom. I never voice these thoughts to my sisters, and my sisters have never voiced these thoughts to me. The doctors and social worker have reminded Mom repeatedly that she can change her mind at any time. The last thing the doctor will do before administering the injection is ask Mom if she still wishes to receive the medication. The hair on the back of my neck went up when I heard this was part of the protocol. How invasive ... and then, *those are the last words Mom will ever hear*?

It is not so much the *question* as the *timing* of the question. I voiced my concern to the physician when he explained the protocol during a family meeting. I couldn't imagine that particular moment ending with this blunt question, but it's the way the protocol is written, and it's written this way for a reason. There *have* been people who changed their minds at the last moment. There were 16,104 requests for MAID in 2022. Some 3,002 individuals did not complete the program, with 46 of those changing their mind at the moment of injection. *Autonomy and choice should never be taken away as long as we are able.* The protocol will be followed.

Mom is too tired to wash up, so I use a warm washcloth to gently bathe her and tuck her in. I have been sleeping with Mom when she feels up to company. Usually, she welcomes me. We always start out snuggling into each other to soak up every last minute we can spend together. I can see that Mom is completely exhausted, but we both agree it has been a wonderful day. By the water. In the sun.

Chapter Six: Cosmos

Sorting through ancient fossil treasures. "Making a memory" are the words Mom loves to use. "Girls, let's make a memory," and the adventure would begin.

One such adventure happened when my daughter Stephanie and her bestie Missy, who was one of Mom's honorary granddaughters, accompanied me on a visit to Mom's place. It was the summer of 1996 and Mom would have been fifty-six years old—four years younger than I am now. Stephanie was twenty-eight years old. We were returning from a rousing game of bingo and had stopped for tea and doughnuts from Tim Hortons. Driving west on Highway 401, we were listening to the radio as we sipped our tea. The 401 is a major highway that runs through the province of Ontario from the Detroit/Windsor border to the Ontario/Quebec border. When the DJ announced that Ontario had just made it legal for women to go topless in public, Mom's eyes got big and round. The girls saw it in the rearview mirror. *We all recognized that look.* It usually came right before one of Mom's almost-crossing-the-line-but-not-quite ideas that might or might not end in some near-miss.

I remember it like this. "Girls, let's make a memory! Off with your tops! Take your bras off too. Let's celebrate!" The tea and doughnuts spilled off to the side as we bared our chests and put the windows down so we could feel the wind caress our skin. With breasts swinging in all their glory, we laughed so hard it was impossible to be self-conscious. Mom loved to have fun, and we all loved to have fun with her.

It's four in the morning when Mom nudges me awake for a snack. Her nightstand is always filled with candy. She rotates her favorites. There are salty snacks and sweet snacks. There are hard candies and soft toffees. Tonight, she removes a few triangles of the white cheese she loves from the top drawer where her pills are kept. Smiling sleepily, I let myself wake up halfway and morph into the younger version of me who would beg for Mom to tell us stories. We didn't want her to read us books. We wanted to hear her stories.

Tonight, they sound different than I remember them as a child, and I realize my listening is being filtered through my life experience. Sixty years of living interprets information differently than the ears of a child. I have lived long enough to know that sometimes life is really hard, and sometimes life

Chapter Six: Cosmos

is really easy, and then there are all the moments in-between. We do our best. Mom did her best. *I release a lifelong sense of responsibility for Mom's mental, physical, and emotional well-being.* She is the mother. I am the daughter. I let my mother tell me stories as I take my time unwrapping the cheese. We are like night-blooming plants who rely on nocturnal pollinators. Some of these stories I have never heard before. I recognize them as gifts that will keep me connected to my mother. I want my daughter to know these stories.

Cosmos flowers are annuals and live for one season. They are grown from seeds, unlike perennials that return year after year and grow from roots. I am putting the garden to rest, but I cannot take out these last colorful remnants of summer. I will wait for the first frost and let nature take its course. This is what we had hoped would be the case for Mom. Like a flower in the first frost, Mom's system would recognize it was time to let go, and her physical body would fall away on its own. This is less and less possible in the current environment of health care. I have rerun this scenario in my head many times over the years. What if Mom had *not* been transferred to a hospital where it was possible for her to have open-heart surgery back in 2000? She would have died at age sixty.

Now, I want Mom to be freed from her shackled body that won't let her work in her garden, *and* I want her to live forever. I want her to have a giant heart attack and leave quickly so we don't have to go through with MAID. I don't want her to have a stroke. A stroke could prevent Mom from confirming her consent right before she receives the medication. There are moments when these competing wants are too much to think about, so I turn my attention back to the cosmos.

Leaving the cosmos in the ground for now will give the seeds a chance to scatter. The flower head consists of an outer ring of ray florets that encircle an inner ring of disc florets. The ray florets or petals are notched and frilly, giving just the slightest appearance of tiny pleats. The petals are soft pinks and reds and saturated hues of raspberry. Some are white with just a hint of color, but they all have the same butter-yellow center. The reproductive heart of the flower. A grouping of smaller green leaves sits on top of the stem and just beneath the flower head.

Chapter Six: Cosmos

The sepal protects the petals during the bud phase of growth and supports the full flower head when the plant matures.

Most of the time it feels like we are all doing this together. Each one of us a vital part of Mom's support system along with the minister, the physician, the nurse, the respiratory therapist, and the pharmacist. Together we form a strong sepal that holds up the flower head. Life has prepared all of us for this moment. The physician is retired. He believes wholeheartedly in MAID, as does the nurse, the minister, and everyone else who volunteers their time for MAID participants and their families. Cosmos leaves are the color of healthy spring grass and have a very distinct lacelike quality. They bring a unique texture to the garden, the way we each bring a unique texture to this time with Mom and with each other. Texture is important and something Mom considers in her plant choices.

All of us are needed for this moment. Some of the cosmos are wilted and discolored. I begin to deadhead these by pinching the flower head off the stem, letting my thumb and index fingers become my garden tools. Everything in nature is reflected in life.

Everything in life appears to be reflected in nature. Do these flowers feel pain when I make the pinch? In my late teens, I was introduced to Kirlian photography through brilliant images of leaves that appeared to be surrounded by a halo of light. At first glance I was sure I was witnessing their aura or energy field. I had no doubt that everything in life was imbued with light, and I didn't question the veracity of the science. In fact, when anything has been intentionally filled with electricity and is then exposed to electrified air, there is a chemical response that results in light. I earned a Bachelor of Science degree in nursing from Ball State University. I graduated with a 4.0 at the top of my class. I trust science *and* I have always secretly hoped the science was wrong. Holding these two contradictory beliefs at the same time is called *cognitive dissonance* and it looks something like this:

"It's a leaf, it can't feel pain." *Or...*

"It's a leaf with its own aura and energy field. Maybe it can feel pain."

"I am relieved the cocktail of medications will prevent Mom from suffering when she dies." *Or...*

"How in the hell can anyone really know that except those who have died?"

Chapter Six: Cosmos

You can deadhead with scissors, but I prefer the tactile experience of touching the plant with the thousands of sensory nerves that end in the tips of my fingers and allow me to know the world through touch. I never wear gloves. I dig my hands right into the dirt. Mom taught me to pinch just above the first set of full healthy leaves. If I want the plant to bush out, I pinch further down the stem to force growth lower on the stem and prevent the plant from becoming spindly.

We are forcing growth as a family right now by meticulously deadheading anything that might cause our connection, our love, or our support to show up as spindly. We are growing a luscious, thick, fertile stalk to support our families and to support Mom's transition. *I am a daughter, but I am also a mother.* While I will be thick in the grieving process, I will still need to be present for my daughter, who will also be thick in the grieving process. I am growing that ability now.

Soft watercolor petals painted in a loose stroke convey the essence of the delicate lacy leaves and movement of cosmos flowers. Mom dabbled with oil paints when she was younger, but once she discovered watercolors, that became her preferred medium. Mom's curiosity merged with her natural talent and she explored many different mediums over the years. All of them self-taught. She showed me that I could be an artist.

Right now, she has my sisters and me knitting hats and scarves for her three adult children and their spouses, her seven grandchildren, and her six great-grandchildren. This qualifies as one of Mom's *making a memory* activities. We are all knitting. Mom adds knit and purl stitches to each woolly creation so her energy can infuse these scarves. Like leaves photographed using the Kirlian technique, Mom wants her love to show up like light surrounding each knit and each purl. For Mom, this feels like a way to forever wrap her arms around each one of us. She is not interested in science. She is interested in leaving her light as a reminder of her love.

Mom is an artist. I am an artist. My daughter is an artist. It is a way of being as much as a choice. I have heard it said that artists give as much attention to the space *between* the objects as they give to the objects themselves, and sometimes even more. This perspective is useful when a sense of helplessness

Chapter Six: Cosmos

tries to wrap around my psyche like a creeping vine. There is little that can be done to alter Mom's health *and* there are endless possibilities for painting these last days with Mom using a palette of colors that reflect back to her the richness of her life.

There were long Sunday drives in our tan 1967 Ford Country Squire station wagon. This classic with its wooden panels had a back, a very-back and a very-very-back section. When we were children, my brother—the youngest of four—always sat in the front seat between my parents. My sisters and I took turns getting the coveted spot at the very-very back, where it felt like you were tucked into a secret hidden fort that also boasted a picture window! Here, you could hunker down and become invisible. Brown bags of penny candy, Archie comic books, and *Teen Beat* magazines were shuffled back and forth as we pored over the latest Donny Osmond and David Cassidy sightings.

When Mom saw something she wanted to sketch, we pulled over. It might be a grouping of trees, an old farmhouse, or an interesting barn found on a random country road. Port Stanley is a small fishing and tourist village on the shores of Lake Erie. Our

Sunday drives often culminated with a stop at Shaw's Dairy. Back then, this was the mecca of all ice cream shops. Spilling through the entrance door, a long white cooler ran the entire length of the shop. Dozens of buckets of ice cream in every flavor and color of the rainbow filled the cooler. Most often, we would have to take a number, which was a thrill all its own for the lucky one who got to pull the tag.

I don't think any of us minded this wait, which gave us time to think about our choice. I loved chocolate, but one day I decided to try licorice *and it was exquisite.* I have learned from experience that choosing something different can be both disarming and rewarding. There are many ways to die. We think we don't have a choice. That somehow it is out of our control. The truth is, from the minute we are born, every second of every minute of every day we are stepping toward the reality that one day *we will die.* This experience with Mom is reminding me of the importance of paying attention to which flavors I choose and why. There is nothing complacent about this journey.

Cosmos make excellent cut flowers that can last up to five days in a vase. I don't recognize the cut-

Chapter Six: Cosmos

glass vase I have filled with water. I found it in the mishmash of glassware in Mom's kitchen cabinet. My sisters and I have gifted her multiple sets of dishes, glassware, mugs, and silverware over the years, but they always seemed to disappear. It is likely that my younger brother found this vase in someone's pile of discarded household items.

I have always been pragmatic about death. Fifteen years of nursing with a good chunk of that spent in critical care units put death right in front of me on a regular basis. Just because we *can* do something with medical technology doesn't mean we *should* do it. Hospital ethics committees are tasked with allocating costly and sometimes scarce resources. I have cared for patients who wanted to die. Some who *longed* to die. There was one man in particular who *begged* to die. In this case, it was the family who could not let go. The attending physician sided with the family. The patient felt helpless and hopeless, and I felt helpless and hopeless to help him.

I am so thankful we have been able to have these frank discussions with Mom and with each other. I have clearly stated my wishes for healthcare interventions in a legal document that both my husband

and my daughter have copies of. I have given them the legal authority to make these decisions for me if ever I am not able. Being here with Mom has cemented the importance of these difficult conversations. *I believe we often confuse the experience of dying with the experience of being the one left behind to grieve.* We lay our woundedness over the one who is dying and assume they are feeling the same way, but they are two different experiences.

When someone we love dies, it can feel like *we* might die or we might wish we *could* die, but we don't. When I worked in hospitals, I tried to be present when I knew death was imminent. I considered it a privilege for my presence to be a safe, quiet space for this profound transition. Many nurses feel this way. *We become more comfortable with death as we experience more death.* I have witnessed how individuals moving closer to death often appear to relax into the transition. Their energy shifts from holding on to release, emotionally and physiologically. This is especially true when the person feels safe and physically cared for. It is not true when the person is struggling for a breath or tensing due to pain.

Chapter Six: Cosmos

We have the means with modern medicine to experience a peaceful death. As we learn to accept death as a normal phase of life, we free ourselves to give the one who is leaving permission. Our focus shifts from advocating for ourselves to advocating for the *one who is dying*. We are quick to talk about the *miracle of life* when an infant enters this world. I believe the *miracle of death* carries the same weight and mystery.

Some of us wait to die surrounded by family, and some of us prefer to die alone. The ethical struggles of modern-day medicine hit close to home when my beloved mother-in-law suffered a large ruptured cerebral aneurism that left very little chance for meaningful recovery. Working at the hospital where she was admitted, I arrived in the emergency department shortly after she was brought in by ambulance. "She has a living will stating she does not want to be kept alive by machinery in the advent of a catastrophic event," I informed the neurologist. I knew how fast life-sustaining measures could be initiated. This was clearly a catastrophic event. Still, she was admitted to the intensive care unit and placed on multiple life-support devices. Having survived a near-fatal heart attack years earlier, she had benefited greatly from medical technology, but by this time, she felt she had lived long enough. *She felt it enough to put it in writing.*

While I was conversing with the neurologist, the intensivist was on the phone convincing her husband that she would feel hunger without a feeding tube. At that time, living wills were just being implemented and talked about. Most people did not have one. In the beginning, they were not always followed if the family objected. What qualified as a catastrophic event was not always as clear as it is now, yet even today there are court battles over the right to die. Most physicians are trained to save lives, not to let people die.

As a family we begged for life support to be removed. It had been days with no signs of consciousness. The CT scan showed half of her cerebrum was in essence already dead. After several days and some difficult conversations, the neurologist agreed to meet us in the ICU to remove life support. There was a lot to undo: a ventilator was breathing for her, a nasogastric tube was preventing her from aspirating the contents of her stomach into her lungs, a feeding

Chapter Six: Cosmos

tube was delivering nutrition in liquid form, a catheter collected her urine, cardiac monitors recorded and beeped alarms with every aberrant heart signal, a pulse oximeter cued the nurses and doctors when to draw more labs and when to titrate the ventilator, cables from the EEG machine protruded from her thick snow-white hair, and a cocktail of synthesized pharmaceuticals sustained her blood pressure.

I stood there on that morning with two of her daughters waiting for the neurologist, who would later apologize to us for not honoring her wishes. As a family we not only said goodbye, but "We love you. We're okay. You've got this. Take flight" … *and she did.* Minutes before we were to remove life support, she went into a lethal heart arrhythmia that even the machines could not reverse. My memories of this moment are visceral. Goose bumps erupted on my arms as I watched her eyes open wide. They shone brightly and radiated pure joy. There were no signs of fear as she flew out of her physical body and stepped into the next version of herself that morning. There was no holding her back. The essence of this sweet spirit left as her body finalized the physiological processes.

This event changed the way I view death in a profound way that I have shared with patients, families, and friends who were facing death and felt fearful. *Death* occurs when the vital organs that support life in our physical body cease to function. *Grief* is the process of reorganization and integration as our hearts and our minds and our spirits learn to live with space that was not there before.

Don't confuse my stoicism in writing with lack of compassion. For close to a year before Mom decided to investigate MAID, her suffering and discomfort slowly but steadily escalated. Most of our phone calls were spent with her crying out her tears and frustration. She sounded hopeless. She expressed hopelessness. Mom had tried every medical intervention the doctors recommended and every nonmedical intervention her family and friends recommended to ease the myriad of symptoms that plagued her. At seventy-nine years old with multiple health issues, it was not practical or feasible to consider a heart transplant, or in Mom's case a heart and at least one lung.

After so many of these calls, it was clear that Mom's quality of life had slipped away. Even her passion for painting could no longer distract her from the pain. One day I said to her, "You know, Mom, you live in a country where you don't have to suffer. You live in a country where you have a choice. I want you to know that I fully support you exploring your choices." And so the conversation had begun.

After arranging the cosmos flowers in the crystal vase, I turn my attention to the yellow snapdragons still blooming prolifically in the garden. Yellow is Mom's favorite color, and these snapdragons will bring a smile to her face. I add them to the vase along with some anemones that add an airy and playful feel to the mix. A few daisies and some black-eyed Susans complete the arrangement. Mom will wake up to the fragrances and colors of her beautiful flowers.

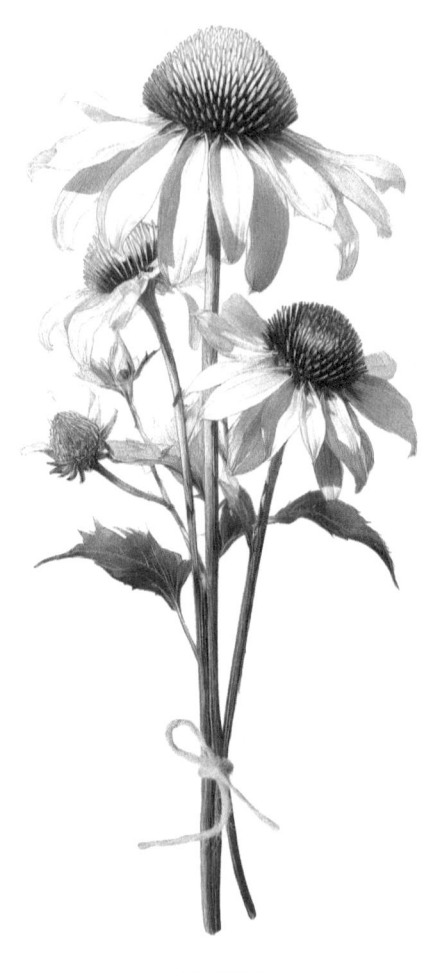

Echinacea purpurea
Common Name – Purple Coneflower

Many of these petals are now shriveled but remain attached to the cone. Even in their shriveled state, the soft colors of the petals give evidence of what once was. So it is with Mom.

Chapter Seven

Purple Coneflower

Journal entry October 15, 2020. This morning, I woke with the devil knocking at my door. "I'm not good enough. Mom doesn't love me. I am unlovable." Oh boy, where did this come from? I thought to call Pete and cry on his shoulder, but really, I don't need to spill this on anyone. I don't want Pete to worry about me. I have learned to notice and feel sensations without reacting to them off the cuff through meditation and movement. Use it, Theresa. Thirty-one days until November 15.

Hiding in plain sight in our gardens, pharmaceuticals pose as leaves, petals, sap, roots, and stems. Many gardeners are aware of the common herbs used for cooking and teas, but few of us are versed in the medicinal bounty growing in our gardens. Baby boomers were the first ones to grow up with antibiotics and rapid growth in the field of medicine. Several generations later, medicine still feels like it is just getting started. What is touted as a panacea one moment is dismissed the next. *It's complicated.*

My Nona was raised in Italy during the generation when antibiotics were discovered. It was 1928. It would be ten more years before they became widely available for market in 1938. At that time the focus was on *living longer*. We were nowhere near the current Right to Die issues. Nona shared the folk remedies she had learned from her mother with our mother. Mom shared what she learned with us. Hot mustard plasters for chest colds, garlic-infused steam for congestion, and warm clove oil for earaches were always Mom's first line of defense.

Echinacea purpurea, whose common name is purple coneflower, is a well-known member of the secret pharmacy. Mom's patch of coneflowers has doubled every year since she planted them four years ago. We all have some of her coneflowers in our own gardens. These hardy perennials developed their strength by adapting to life on the prairies. If you look closely, you will see the stem and leaves are covered with small white hairs that provide shade and break up the drying winds that can frequent the prairie.

My grandmother's mother would have watched her family and friends—including babies, teenagers, adults, and elders—die at the hands of bacteria that became easy to treat once antibiotics became available. Now, these same bacteria have morphed into resistant strains due to overexposure to some of these antibiotics. MRSA (methicillin-resistant Staphylococcus aureus) is a current superbug that is killing patients while they are hospitalized for unrelated ailments. The CDC or Centers for Disease Control reports that one in thirty-one patients will contract a *nosocomial* (hospital-acquired) infection. None of this was known when Mom's generation in particular became enamored with exotic cocktails of pharmaceuticals.

It seemed there was a cure for *everything.* Even conditions we were not aware we had. Antibiotics flowed freely, and it wasn't until years later that we realized the danger of creating resistant bacteria like MRSA. Here, the conversation becomes cloudy. Like an aquatic plant lying on the muddy bottom of murky waters, we are trying valiantly to suss out the moralities of modern medical interventions. An intervention is called a miracle when it saves the life of anyone we love. That same intervention becomes fodder for grief and anger when our loved one experiences an adverse effect. Interventions are not dispersed equally in our society. These days natural remedies seem impotent next to the powerful drugs that have been developed over the last 150 years. We want a pill for everything that ails us, and we want it to work quickly. *It's complicated.*

We all adapt and grow under the influence of our environments. When the conditions are right, we grow strong and vital and we thrive. When an important building block is missing, we still grow, but our foundation suffers. Mom's foundation has never been strong. She was always reluctant to share her personal story with us, as if telling us her story would make it our story, but over the years we drew bits and pieces out of her. She told me once about daily rations of soda biscuits on short stints back with her birth family. When fruit *was* available, the children were given the peels to eat while her father ate the fruit. I have always believed Mom's negligible grip on health was a result of her poor nutrition and lack of nurturing while she was still develop-

Chapter Seven: Purple Coneflower

ing. Like a plant that reaches for the light through a crack in the sidewalk, these circumstances never dampened Mom's determination to create a meaningful life. *Instead, they left their insidious imprint on Mom's tenuous health.*

Coneflowers spread via rhizomes. As long as there is the right light and open space, rhizomes will proliferate or multiply indefinitely to fill the space and then some. This is somewhat akin to our vascular system. With the right conditions, we will continue to repair and regenerate new blood vessels that help nourish different areas as needed. *We are wired to survive.* Right now, these coneflowers look faded and tired, like Mom looks these days. Like I feel right now.

Mom is still sleeping, and I take myself out to the garden in hopes the healing energy of the plants and earth and sun will send this devil on its way. Mom loves to share the knowledge she has learned about her plants. "Native Americans used the root of the coneflower, dear. They used it for headaches, toothaches, sore throats, and even rattlesnake bites." As a child and young adult, I let a lot of this information go in one ear and out the other. Now, I am eager to soak up every word Mom speaks. I want to hear *all* of her stories. All of her crazy ideas. I would not have been surprised to find Mom had dried and powdered echinacea roots in an attempt to test their properties. I was used to Mom being curious.

These coneflowers stand about three feet tall on strong, tough, greenish-brown ribbed stems covered in very fine white hairs. They have a rough texture like sandpaper. The lance-shaped leaves are covered in the same small white hairs. The base of the leaf is wide and narrows to form a point at the tip. I notice the leaves are larger at the base of the stem and decrease in size and quantity as they move up the stem. The leaves are singlets instead of the pairs we often see on other plants.

The major vein and secondary veins are prominent on these rich dark-green serrated leaves. The disc florets standing erect in the center always grab my attention when I am in the presence of coneflowers. Looking closely, I can see they are green at their base and gradually transition into vibrant, orange-tinted yellow spikes that form the convex or cone-shaped center. This is where the *cone* part of the name originates. The disc florets arrange themselves in Fibonacci spirals, which are patterns based on a simple number sequence found over and over again in nature, in human anatomy, and in the cosmos.

We are all connected. I can't resist touching the disc florets with my finger. I expect to feel a prick, but they move easily under gentle pressure. They feel strong and soft at the same time. This is how we all feel right now, my mom, my sisters, and me. The disc florets bend slightly but return to their upright stance when I take my finger away. The ray florets or outer petals appear frail and delicate against the strong stem and leaves. These are a pale lavender pink color with darker hues bordering on magenta coloring faint vertical lines on daisy-shaped petals.

Many of these petals are now shriveled but remain attached to the cone. Even in their shriveled state, the soft colors of the petals give evidence of what once was. So it is with Mom. I look with *softer eyes* to see what she needs these days and I listen to the *space* between her words and to her silence to hear what she can no longer say, but she is still my mom. She is still my teacher.

When echinacea is first blooming, the ray florets lie horizontal to the cone. With time, these petals begin to orient toward the earth and give the cone even more prominence. The cone is the pollination center. The ray florets have evolved their color to attract butterflies and other pollinators. I will check with Mom before I do anything with this plant. It is personal preference whether to cut these back or leave them standing so the birds might enjoy the seeds throughout the long winter.

There is a light tapping on the front window, and I look up to see Mom. Still in her pajamas with bed-tousled hair, she has gotten herself out of bed and into her chair. She has made herself a cup of tea and a piece of toast with butter. I take all of this in when I enter the house, along with the fact that Mom's walker is still in her bedroom. She is stubborn. She always has been. I wonder if this is a trait she developed to survive years of neglect: to help her manage four children when she was but a child herself, to continue in a marriage that did not thrive but at least provided the basic needs of food, clothing, and shelter. Maybe this is part of her inherited Irish DNA. I suspect it to be a little bit of all these things. The impact of *nature versus nurture* has provided rich fodder for social scientists.

"Theresa, you're working too hard. The garden looks great. Come sit and have a tea with me." Her

Chapter Seven: Purple Coneflower

mother-love brings a smile to my face, and I walk into the kitchen to make my tea. There is echinacea tea in Mom's kitchen cupboard with a picture of purple coneflowers on the box. The label proclaims this tea "fires up the immune system." An asterisk directs me to the small disclaimer at the bottom. "These statements have not been evaluated by the Food & Drug Administration. This product is not intended to diagnose, treat, cure, or prevent any disease."

I choose good old black Lipton tea. I make it like Mom's. Strong and hot with lots of milk. We were very young when Mom taught my sisters and me how to make her version of a perfect cup of tea. She could always tell if we grew impatient and didn't let the water come to a rolling boil before we poured it into the cup. In those cases, we would do it again starting from scratch. The milk *(never cream for tea)* goes into the cup first, and the tea is poured into the milk. British rituals may be a distant memory in Canada these days, but I suspect this is a leftover from the English.

"How are you feeling this morning, Mom? Where is your walker?" She looks at me defiantly. "I hate that stupid thing. My oxygen cord gets all caught up in it. I can't carry anything. I walk better just hanging on to things as I go." "But, Mom, I don't want you to fall. I am here to help you. I can make your tea. I can help you with your walker." She responds, "I may be dying in days, but I am alive right now, and this morning I can make my own tea."

"OK, Mom." I cringe when I hear the word *dying* and I hope Mom doesn't notice. My nervous system can handle transformation or transmutation or taking flight or even taking a very long sleep, but there is a finality to the word dying that I have yet to make peace with.

I notice Mom's ankles are overflowing her slippers this morning. They are swollen all the time but more than usual this morning. Her legs appear shiny and pale with jagged blue veins that lie close to the surface of her translucent skin. Unlike the stem of the coneflower that is *covered* in fine white hairs, there are but a few fine white hairs on Mom's legs. Hair loss, shiny skin, pallor … these are all signs of Mom's advanced peripheral arterial disease. Right now, her feet look purple and dusky. I let myself take in this tired, pale version of Mom. I have seen this version many times in my life, but I can sense this time is different. I remind myself that she *should* look tired and pale. That is why

Chapter Seven: Purple Coneflower

I am here—that is why we are going through with the MAID program. Plants need water and the nutrients from the soil. We need blood flow that is rich in oxygen.

I use my finger to see how much *edema* or fluid has collected in Mom's legs. Pressing it gently into her ankle, it leaves a deep indentation that does not bounce back. When I listen to her lungs with my stethoscope I hear *rattling*, or signs of fluid in the bases of her lungs. Her congestive heart failure is roiling up. I decide to give her a Lasix pill. This medication acts as a diuretic and will clear some of the extra fluid she is holding by making her pee more. The fluid is backing up in Mom's system because the right side of her heart is no longer pumping effectively.

The left side of the heart pumps blood out to our body. If the left side fails (for any of various reasons), back pressure will cause excess fluid to accumulate in the lungs. That excess fluid is what I hear when I listen to her lungs. The right side of the heart (specifically, the right atria) is where the electrical impulse arises that regulates heart rate and rhythm. Mom has atrial fibrillation, which causes the atria or upper chambers of the heart to fire chaotically rather than in a normal steady rhythm. In a healthy heart, the atria pump extra blood into the ventricles immediately before the ventricles contract. This adds about 20% extra to our cardiac output. When we lose this extra kick due to atrial fibrillation, the heart is not nearly as effective.

All of this contributes to heart failure, with the eventual collection of excess fluid in our lungs and in our legs. This chaotic random firing does not allow for efficient filling in the lower chambers (ventricles), and consequently the lower chambers cannot function normally.

I haven't worked as a cardiac nurse for twenty years now, but this knowledge is embedded in my brain from long days in cardiac units. Congestive heart failure gone unchecked feels as if you are drowning—because simply put, you *are* drowning.

Still, I feel nervous about making these decisions for Mom. Once again, my thoughts go to all the caregivers who are in the same spot as I am right now and have no medical background to support their decisions. I decide to record the medication and call the nurse so she knows what is going on. Mom hates to take Lasix. Her energy will be used up making multiple trips to the bathroom to pee out the extra fluid. We have borrowed

Chapter Seven: Purple Coneflower

a commode for nighttime use, but she still prefers to get to her bathroom during the day.

Most days Mom has given up on wearing shoes, even when we venture out. Mom loved her shoes. Almost as much as she loved her purses. We have donated most of her shoes, boots, and purses by now. Slippers are more comfortable and let her ankles spill into the space around them without the restriction that shoes impose. *I am filled with contradiction.* I wish we didn't have all these potent drugs and yet I am grateful for the Lasix that will ease her breathing and the workload of her heart. Without medical interventions and drugs, Mom would have died long ago.

"I am working with the coneflowers this morning, Mom. Is there anything special I need to know?" She asks me to leave them standing and clean up around them. "Birds love the seeds in the center. They will eat them in the winter when food may be hard to find. We'll just let the petals fall to the ground. Put some mulch around them if they need it, dear." "OK, Mom." I knew this would be her preference. *Mom won't let anyone or any creature go hungry.* The devil may still be lurking in the distance, but for the moment my heart is soft again.

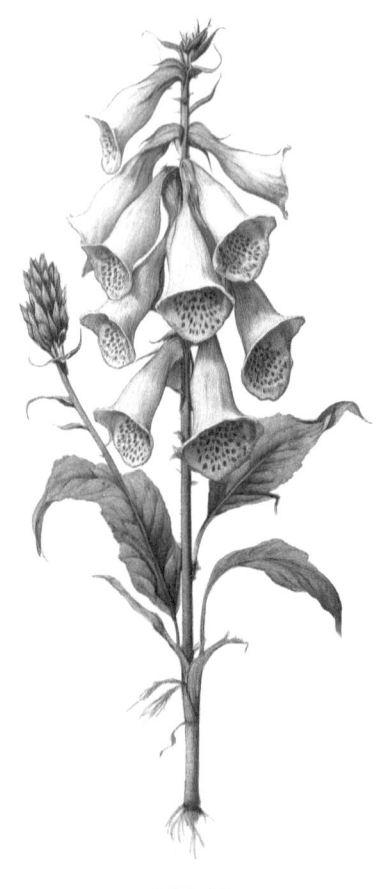

Digitalis
Common Name – Foxglove

My mind is wandering and wondering. What did people do a hundred years ago when they developed heart failure? Would they have brewed a tea using the leaves of the foxglove plant based on folklore gleaned from their ancestors or the local healer?

Chapter Eight

Foxglove

Journal entry October 21, 2020. Today was my sixty-first birthday. It was exceptionally warm and sunny and a perfect day to putter in the garden. Mom said she wanted to make a memory and make it special for me. She gave me her last piece of apple pie and the last of the ice cream. Two things my mother is very fond of. A way for her to show her mother-love. I don't know what I thought sixty-one would feel like ... but the longer I live, the more I realize a number is simply a number. I can look back and say I have lived sixty-one years filled with adventure and boredom and joy and sadness and everything in-between. We create a life with the bits and pieces that land in front of us. I have done my best. Mostly, I am grateful to be here right now with Mom and my sisters. Twenty-five days until November 15.

Foxglove is a potent medicinal plant. The biennial varieties bloom every other year while the true perennial varieties bloom every year. Foxgloves bloom in spring and summer; if they are deadheaded, they may bloom yet again in late summer. Standing as a testament that summer is over and fall has arrived, the foxgloves in Mom's garden are past their prime. Mom has left the flower spike of this biennial variety standing. The seedpods are now rust colored and dry, each one filled with hundreds or thousands of seeds that will fall and resow for next season. Mom is letting the *Anemoi* or Greek wind gods decide where the seeds will settle.

My nurse brain remembers that foxglove is also called *digitalis*. I have administered digitalis to hundreds of patients with heart issues over the years. Mom has taken digitalis or digoxin at some point in her adult life. Foxglove is toxic to both humans and animals. Inhaling the pollen can cause adverse reactions in some people, while the fine white hairs that cover the leaves can irritate the skin of others. Long ago this deceivingly beautiful plant earned the name *dead man's bells* or *witch's gloves*, which speaks to the poisonous qualities of foxgloves. In the right

Chapter Eight: Foxglove

dose, digitalis is very useful for specific types of heart failure. Mom had that significant heart attack at the age of sixty. She was one year younger than I am now. The damage was to the left side of her heart.

The left side of your heart is responsible for pumping oxygen-rich blood from the lungs out to the peripheral system. It is the *worker* side of the heart. Ironically, Mom's heart attack was attributed to the use of the drug Vioxx. Remembering this sends me spinning down a rabbit hole and into the quagmire that makes up the pharmaceutical industry.

Mom was prescribed Vioxx for arthritis that increasingly limited her ability to do those things she loved: gardening, knitting, sewing, golfing, and even walking. Her arthritis affected all of her joints. Vioxx was like a miracle drug. Those of you who used it know it was *very* effective in relieving pain. *There is that which we can see and that which we cannot see...* While Vioxx *was* improving the quality of life for thousands with its ability to decrease pain, it was silently increasing the chance of heart attacks by increasing the incidence of blood clots. When a clot forms on plaque that is present in a coronary artery, it can block blood flow through the artery. In some, the clot traveled to the brain, which resulted in a stroke. At the time of its recall, the FDA estimates that Vioxx may have caused 140,000 heart attacks, resulting in an estimated 60,000 deaths.

Vioxx was pulled from the market in 2004 after research showed the strong positive correlation between the use of Vioxx, heart attacks, and strokes. It was already too late for Mom. Monsanto had manufactured Vioxx and enlisted the pharmaceutical company Merck to help market the drug. There was a 4.85-billion-dollar settlement levied against Merck in 2007, but the process of submitting a claim was so difficult and drawn out that many of those affected did not receive a payout. This included Mom. After countless hours spent by Mom and my sister gathering and sorting years' worth of medical records, we were advised there was *one* record missing from the paperwork they had submitted for the claim. When my sister tried to submit it, she was told the window for submissions had closed. What is a heart worth anyway? Mom was literally *heartbroken.*

According to the 2024 *Heart Disease and Stroke Statistics*, heart disease has been the leading cause of death in the United States for a hundred years.

Chapter Eight: Foxglove

As a culture, we have poured our faith into modern pharmaceuticals and we have come to believe and *expect* there is a pill for everything and for everything a pill. We want fast results *and* we don't want to give up the lifestyle choices that have let heart disease run rampant: cigarette smoking, excessive alcohol, poor nutrition, and lack of exercise. If we put the same amount of faith in nutrition and exercise, quit smoking, and quit or decreased alcohol consumption, we could greatly reduce our risk of heart attacks and stroke.

Mom's generation grew up never questioning what the doctor ordered. As a nurse, I cared for patients who had no idea what medications they were taking, and more importantly, why they were taking them. Great strides have been made in providing this information, but there is still ample room for improvement. If cognitively capable, we should know *why* we are taking a drug, any *interactions* that may occur with other drugs or supplements, how certain foods can alter how we *metabolize* the drug, and the *side effects* of the drug.

My mind is wandering and wondering. What did people do a hundred years ago when they developed heart failure? Would they have brewed a tea using the leaves of the foxglove plant based on folklore gleaned from their ancestors or the local healer? Dosing is an issue. How do you know exactly how much digitalis you are ingesting when you munch down a leaf or make a tea? We probably died faster and younger.

Digitalis or digoxin is a chemical known as a *cardiac glycoside.* Digoxin helps the heart pump slower so the heart chambers have time to fill. It helps the heart pump stronger to move the blood into the system and decrease the workload for the compromised cardiac muscle. Digitalis was first isolated from the foxglove plant in 1930 but was not approved by the Food and Drug Administration until 1954. It took *twenty-four* years for this drug to make it to market and to those who might benefit from it. In 2024 we are being told *artificial intelligence* will soon take over clinical trials for the efficacy and safety of new pharmaceuticals. A computer program will simulate every possible scenario in hours rather than years, and new drugs will make it to market in record time. The information we live by now will become folklore in the future, and the cycles of life will continue. *Integration and disintegration.*

Chapter Eight: Foxglove

Deep purple spots ringed with white appear on the inside bottom petal of the tubular foxglove flowers. These meticulous miniature canvases are not the result of haphazard brush strokes at the hands of nature but serve a greater purpose in attracting bumblebees, which are the main pollinators for this plant. The pendulous flowers can reach two and a half inches in length and rest on a central spike that shoots out of a thick spiral of coarse leaves called the rosette.

In the first year, biennials often form a rosette where they absorb and store nutrients and energy for the second year when the flower spike will appear. A foxglove rosette displays large rough leaves with prominent veins and serves as a ground-level centerpiece for the flower spike that will shoot out of the center in the second year. A single stem or spike can hold twenty to eighty flowers in shades of white, light pink, purple, and yellow. There are five individual petals that fuse together to form the tubular flowers or corollas. Each flower rests on its sepal, which protects the young buds and later supports the mature flowers.

Nature will often make a toxic plant unappealing to deter both humans and wildlife from accidental poisoning, but the old-fashioned splendor of the foxglove appears more like an invitation. The botanical name *digitalis* means finger. An old wives' tale recounts the story of fox wearing these finger hats on their paws to dampen their sound when hunting prey. I imagine a fox trotting around in purple foxglove booties and smile.

Each Friday Mom receives her medications for the week in several *blister packs* from the local pharmacy. These are a godsend as Mom is on so many medications right now that even I feel overwhelmed by the volume despite my medical background. There are pills that make her heart beat harder and slower. There are pills that help her kidney function by increasing her urine flow. There are pills that lower her blood pressure by dilating the arteries. There are pills that reduce acid reflux and pills that help with constipation. There are pills for her restless legs and pills for depression and anxiety. *There are pills that purportedly help with pain.* This has become a messy quagmire as opiate addiction has surged over the years. While Mom's pain has continued to increase, her ability to procure pain medication has become more and more difficult.

Chapter Eight: Foxglove

Each visit to her doctor is preceded with fear that her pain medication will be reduced or canceled. When my brother was still alive, I know he was buying her Percocet on the streets, and I didn't stop him. We were all breaking right along with Mom as she cried her suffering all over us. Now that she is officially dying, we have been delivered enough narcotics to put down a horse if needed. Why now? The last few years of Mom's life have been usurped by pain and poor pain management. She has cried to be heard and seen by those in the medical profession. Not long ago she looked at me and said, "Old people are invisible. I am invisible."

Herein lies the conundrum. Mom is taking enough medications to keep her alive, but not enough to give her any *quality* of life. My sisters and I have done our best to intervene for Mom. She is lucky to have us as there are many in the same situation who are alone. Mom has always been considered a *noncompliant* patient. A label assigned to those who for one reason or another do not follow their prescribed medical regimen. Over the years I have arrived at Mom's house to find blister packs that had been opened but not completely emptied or simply forgotten entirely. This was Mom's attempt to manage the side effects on her own. Her inherent lack of trust in the medical system has grown, even though she has spent much of her life dependent on this system.

There is a shortage of primary care doctors in her area, and we have struggled to find her not just a competent doctor, but *any* doctor who is taking new patients. The politics are not helpful. When a physician sees someone is already on narcotics, they are reluctant to take them on as a patient because their hands are tied. A doctor who spends a small fortune on a medical education, studies for eight or more years, and starts with a keen desire to heal is now being told what he or she can prescribe, how much they can prescribe, and who they can prescribe it to by those who control the money. This is a complex issue. I have walked both sides of the tracks as a nurse, a nurse case manager, a patient, and as the family member of a patient. There is no easy answer. I believe it is a *system* issue. We need systems in place that support both the needs of the medical professionals and the patients. There is often a feeling on both sides that we are frantically treading water. *Sometimes drowning feels like the only alternative.*

Chapter Eight: Foxglove

I turn my attention back to the foxgloves. The seed pods have split open and are empty. Potentially thousands of seeds have scattered in the garden, with the promise of more foxglove spikes heavy with their old-fashioned medicinal tubular flowers in the spring. I cut down the dead flower stems, cut back the rosette, and cover it all with mulch, aware that each plant I put to rest moves me closer to November 15 and Mom's birthday.

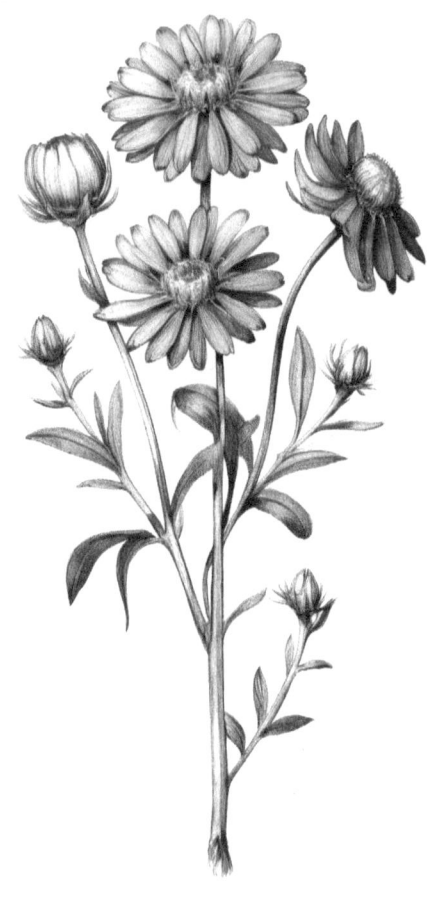

Aster amellus
Common Name – Asters

Aster in Greek means "star." This name fits the star-like configuration the ray petals make. Mom planted these to add some fall color to the garden.

Chapter Nine

Asters

Journal entry October 26, 2020. Several days ago, Mom asked me to take her dog Rosie in to be put to sleep. Rosie is a Pomeranian. She is 14 years old. She is demanding. She is a barker. She has four teeth left and she is not quick to warm up to anyone other than Mom. My sisters and I used to joke about Mom and her psychotic dogs. Rosie and I have history. I can't say that she likes me, but she has hidden in my bag several times for clandestine trips into the hospital to visit Mom. We have an understanding.

 I had offered to bring Rosie home with me, but Mom felt she would struggle with the change and with my dogs Lucy and Lily. We have an appointment with the veterinarian tomorrow at 3:00 p.m. Slowly, Mom has been letting go of things in her own timing and rhythm. I am doing my best not to interfere with this rhythm. The days continue to dissolve faster than the speed it feels we are moving. Twenty days until November 15.

My pace is slowing along with Mom's—like when you hold someone long enough and you begin to breathe in sync with each other. My sisters and I spend afternoons sitting on the couch knitting with Mom. Yes, Mom is still knitting. *We are all still knitting!*

We have begun the process of cleaning and clearing out Mom's belongings. She wants this completed before she leaves. She wants her home staged and ready for sale. She wants to meet the realtor and have everything ready so the For Sale sign can go up in the yard as soon as she is gone. I am down with all of this, but one of my sisters is struggling. For her it feels like we are hastening Mom's death by disposing of her personal belongings before she has left. I have asked Mom to speak with her and help her understand her wishes. I am caught between Mom's wishes and my sisters' emotions. Here is the thing with families—we all have our own individual timing, and sometimes one person's timing is on a collision course with another person's timing. As November 15 grows closer, our hearts are raw and easily bruised.

Asters are late-summer-and-fall-blooming perennials. Mom's asters are blue with slender softly

Chapter Nine: Asters

pointed ray petals attached to bright yellow disc centers. They are part of the daisy family. I love blue flowers. Bees love blue flowers too. Asters are some of the last plants standing for the pollinators. I have taken to bringing Mom's gardening book with me when I work in the garden. I am learning and honing my gardening skills between my mom's rich personal experience and her wonderful reference books. She has given me the gardening book *Rodale's Illustrated Encyclopedia of Perennials*. It has been a staple on her bookshelf.

Aster in Greek means "*star*." This name fits the starlike configuration the ray petals make. Mom planted these to add some fall color to the garden. They are planted strategically to hide earlier bloomers like the iris and daylilies that have finished for the season and are now dormant for the winter. I have never had the best luck with asters. Mine always look somewhat bedraggled and lanky, and now I wonder if they are getting enough sun. Mom's asters are full of flower heads. The stems almost reach the height of the picket fence and span an area roughly four feet wide. This is a robust patch. I decide to dig up a clump to transplant in my sister's garden. I can do this now and put them in a temporary pot. Little by little we have been moving plants from Mom's garden to my sister's garden.

Mom has asked me to dig a hole in my sister's garden where we will bury Rosie. She wants it deep enough that no other animals will dig her up. I am to wrap Rosie in her favorite blanket. The one she has always slept on. We have planned another deep dive with the help of some medicinal mushrooms for Sunday if the weather is nice. I want Rosie's final resting place to bring Mom a sense of peace when she sees it. A place of honor in my sister's garden. I have enough time to go over there and prepare the site now. Digging up a big clump of asters, I find a large bucket to put them in. It's not ideal to move plants while they are blooming, as this disrupts the root system and potentially their ability to take up water and nutrients. I do it anyway and take an extra-large dirt ball in hopes the asters won't even notice they have been relocated.

The earth in my sister's garden has been enriched with manure and fertilizer over the forty years they have lived here. It's easy to dig, and I have no problem preparing a nice deep hole for Rosie's body. As I take

Chapter Nine: Asters

in the beauty of these gardens with the sun reflecting off the tall wispy grasses, I feel a pang of sadness and regret that Mom has never had her hands in my garden. She has spent a lot of time over here helping my sister. It is simply a matter of proximity. Mom would have loved to help me if I hadn't lived so far away. We have had many long-distance gardening sessions via Facetime. I will miss walking through my garden with Mom on my phone.

Journal entry October 26, 2020. I need to record this comedy of errors carefully for posterity. Today I took Rosie to the vet to have her euthanized. Mom was very calm as I gathered Rosie and prepared to leave. I think she had been preparing herself for this moment, and quite honestly, I could see that even Rosie's barking was becoming too much for Mom's fragile nervous system. Mom was ticking off the "to do" list in preparation for November 15.

On my way out the door I noticed Mom still had Lil's ashes in a box on the dresser. Lil was Mom's previous psycho dog—a Yorkie who I gave up trying to pet because she turned werewolf on me anytime I approached her. I decided to take Lil and bury her with Rosie. Together, Rosie and I waited in the treatment room. Despite the warm day, goose bumps covered my bare skin. I held Rosie close to my chest swaddled in her favorite blanket. I could do this.

The vet walked in. He was a soft-spoken man who put me at ease with his gentle demeanor. He examined Rosie thoroughly and then looked up at me and asked me why I had come. I was taken by surprise as I thought I had thoroughly explained all of the details when I made the appointment. "This is my mom's dog. My mom is dying on November 15 via the MAID program. She would like Rosie to be euthanized as she is old and very attached to her. She does not believe Rosie could be happy without her."

The vet listened intently, but I could see the smooth skin of his forehead begin to furrow, telling me this might not be as cut-and-dry as I had anticipated. He said he would be back, turned around, and walked out of the room. Whew. He had gone to get the medication. In a few minutes he returned and took Rosie's temperature. I silently questioned why such a thorough exam for a dog that was about to be

Chapter Nine: Asters

put to sleep, but what did I know about the protocol. With soulful eyes, he looked up at me and quietly stated, "I cannot in all good conscience euthanize this dog. Old age is simply not a suitable reason. She is very healthy despite her age and her lack of teeth. I won't charge you for the visit, but I cannot do what you have asked."

Something inside me broke. Everything I had not been able to feel or express since arriving at Mom's poured out of me. The dam burst. Uncontrollable tears streamed down my face as I sobbed and shook and choked out to the doctor that there was no way I could possibly return home to my mother's with Rosie. It would kill her. This decision had been so hard for her to make. Please, please, please, I begged him—please put this dog down.

At this point, rationale was not part of the equation. I would have to kill her myself. I looked at the vet and exclaimed, "I will have to kill her myself. Please don't make me have to kill her myself!" Memories of Mom drowning newborn kittens in a bucket on our farm flooded my thoughts. Could I really drown this dog? Farm life is full of life and death. Animals are cared for and respected, but they are animals. Too many barn cats are too many barn cats. Better they die early, before they realize they are alive. Anthropomorphism is not practiced on a working farm—or at least was not on our working farm. Mom had learned how to survive on a farm from my father's mother, my Nona. They had immigrated from Italy and arrived in Canada with little to get them started. Working a farm they could never afford to own meant nothing was wasted and decisions were based on practicality. This is how Mom learned to drown kittens.

Life is not black-and-white. During the years my parents had their own farm, many foals were born in our birthing stall. My mother spent countless nights during those years sleeping in the cold barn waiting to assist if needed. She never missed a birth and became a midwife in the process.

The receptionist walked into the examining room and placed her hand on my shoulder. "I know someone who would love to adopt Rosie. An older woman who lives alone. She has one small dog, and both of them would love another companion." I looked at her. I couldn't think. I was shaking. I was overwhelmed. I needed air. I needed to hear my husband's voice. I needed to be talked off the cliff. I headed for the door. Even before I stepped outside, I had decided that I would not call my sisters. If I was about to kill Rosie or to not kill Rosie, I didn't want them to carry the burden of this knowledge. I knew we were all barely holding it together despite our brave faces. I called my husband, and his voice—calm and filled with love—guided me back to myself. Back to the present moment. I had been gone for two months. I had been too preoccupied with Mom to realize how much I missed him. I knew I couldn't kill Rosie. Pete knew I couldn't kill Rosie. We decided together on a closed adoption.

At that moment, I looked up and there was my youngest sister walking down the street. "What are you doing? Why are you crying? More importantly, why is Rosie still alive?" she cried. "What are you doing here?" I asked her. Mom had sent her to see what was going on. She felt I had been gone too long with no word and suspected there was a problem. I filled her in on the details. "Shit, shit, shit..." she said. She wrapped her arms around me and our tears morphed into semi-hysterical giggles as we visualized Mom leaving her body only to see Rosie in the arms of a stranger on her way out! Surely, she would curse us for the rest of our lives.

Together we went inside and talked to the receptionist. I made her remove any information regarding my mother or Rosie from their computer system. I watched her do it. I watched her search for Mom's name, and nothing came up. I made her swear an oath of secrecy. I told her in no uncertain terms that Rosie's adoptive mother could not plaster pictures of her cute new furry ball of love all over Facebook, which Mom still frequented to connect with friends. I handed Rosie over along with her favorite blanket. We walked out of the office. I asked my sister to go back to Mom's and tell her that all was well. There had been a bit of a wait, but it had all gone very quickly and peacefully. "Tell her I have gone to bury Rosie and then I will be straight home."

I took Lil and placed her ashes in the hole I had dug for Rosie. With each shovelful of earth, I prayed for grace. I prayed I had done the right thing. I prayed my mom would never find out. I took the beautiful blue asters and carefully watered them into the freshly turned earth. I gathered some large pieces of granite and other indigenous rock and placed them

Chapter Nine: Asters

in a circle to guard the asters and create the illusion of a safe resting place. As I turned around to gather my tools and head for Mom's, a monarch butterfly landed on the asters. I took this to be a sign. All was well. I had done my best.

When I returned home, Mom was anxiously waiting for me. My sister's dog Gaia was curled on her lap. "Thank you, Theresa. Thank you so much, dear. That must have been so hard for you." She held me close. "Yes, Mom, it was hard, but I am OK. Rosie is OK. We are OK." *There is that which we can see and that which we cannot see...*

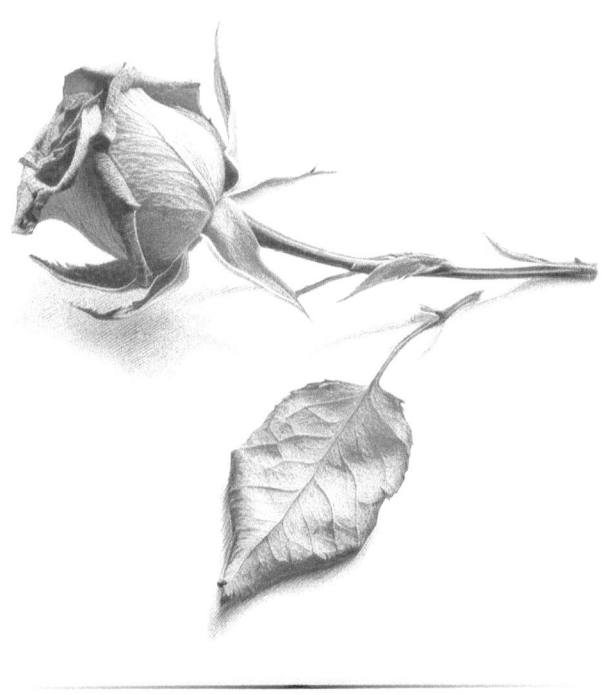

Rosa
Common Name – Roses

At the funeral, the tiny casket was covered with yellow roses. In the baby book is a dried and faded red rose that my father brought to Mom upon learning of Louise's death. This is why there are no roses in Mom's garden. There have never been any roses in Mom's gardens.

Chapter Ten

ROSES

Journal entry October 29, 2020. My sisters and I took Mom on a 150-kilometer road trip to Milton, Ontario. This is the place where all of us were born. I had not been there for fifty years. I was in third grade when my family moved to St. Thomas, Ontario, where my father had found work at the new Ford assembly plant. We were returning to Milton today because Mom wanted to visit the gravesites of her oldest daughter and her youngest daughter, who had both died as infants. Our sisters Louise and Maria. I had never been to these gravesites or to this cemetery. One night in bed in her final weeks, Mom shared this story with me again. I will convey the details as accurately as I can remember them. Seventeen days until November 15.

After meeting the handsome Italian boy at that fateful baseball game, and the whirlwind of falling pregnant, becoming emancipated from the Children's Aid Society, getting married at just seventeen, and moving in with Nona and Nonno and the rest of the extended family, Mom did not have an easy time of it. Morning sickness that morphed into afternoon sickness followed her all through her pregnancy. She was physically tired. She was living in a crowded old farmhouse that reverberated with yelling and shouting in a language she did not understand. One small bathroom downstairs housed the clawfoot tub and rust-stained toilet. My parents lived in the unfinished and unheated attic. Food was stretched. Money was scarce. *Mom was thriving.*

Any doubts about her present state of affairs were diluted by her love for this baby she carried. She was impatient to hold this precious child. Her moment to create the life and the family she had always wanted to be part of lay growing in her belly. She would care for this child the way she had never been cared for. She loved my father and she loved my father's mother. Nona was the closest Mom had come to having a *real* mother. Nona taught her how to cook the food of Italy. To butcher a chicken for dinner. To take that chicken and add onion, celery, carrots, garlic, tomatoes, and greens from the garden

Chapter Ten: Roses

to create an Italian feast. Always there was pasta. A healthy sprinkling of Parmesan cheese added the finishing touch.

Meat hung from strings in the basement. Mom learned how to make the dough for crostoli. A beloved childhood memory for me and an anticipated part of any visit to the farm when we were children was the making of crostoli. Mom learned to roll the dough onto the old oilcloth covering the large kitchen farm table like Nona did. Her hands learned to *feel* the thickness as she rolled; thin enough that you could almost see through it but thick enough for the diagonal cuts that shaped the pastry. She learned to drop the pieces one by one into the spitting oil in the heavy cast iron frying pan. When the pastry turned golden in the center and the edges were just beginning to brown, the crostoli was set to cool on wire racks. A final dusting with powdered sugar added the sweetness. Just writing this makes me pine for one of these childhood treats.

Here is where Mom was introduced to Catholicism. Nona never missed church, and Mom never missed going with her. The small old-fashioned church was filled mostly with Italian immigrants looking to start a new life. For these women, still clothed in the traditional long black dresses of the old life, church was a treasured and familiar landing place for their faith. Their understanding was *visceral* and far outweighed any need-to-know Latin. This was 1958, and the Second Vatican Council had not yet convened. Women covered their heads and Communion was received kneeling at the rail. Only the priest could touch the host as he placed it on your outstretched tongue and the body of Christ dissolved in your mouth.

Sins were confessed in dark wooden confessionals carved with symbols at the back of the church. Old wooden pews creaked and squeaked as the congregation shifted from kneeling to sitting like *the wave* at a football game. Scents of frankincense and myrrh wafted through the air, permeating every surface. Lips murmured automatic replies in a call and response chant between the priest and the parishioners. "In the name of the Father, the Son, and the Holy Spirit. The Lord be with you. And also, with you." These words were long ago imprinted into the memories of the faithful. Rosary beads carefully slipped bead by bead through pairs of entwined

Chapter Ten: Roses

hands as the faithful did penance and prayed away the sins from the previous week.

A liturgical calendar hung in Nona's kitchen and announced the holy days and feast days. Mom learned the customs and rituals of the church. She wanted to be a good Catholic—no, she wanted to be a *great* Catholic. She clung to the belief that suffering was part of life and the hope that embracing her new religion would be the beginning of a brighter future. Louise was born on October 5, 1958, in a small country hospital outside of Milton. She carried an unspoken promise of family and love. Mom said she was so beautiful. So vibrant. So completely alive. A miracle. The nurses and visitors said she was too beautiful. Mom used to put emphasis on this when she would tell the story … *everyone said she was too beautiful.*

Mom had her very own child to love like she herself had never been loved. In those days a stay in the hospital for up to a week followed childbirth. During that week Mom held Louise as often as she could. She fought with the nurses when they came to take her away. She fed and bathed Louise and learned how to care for this precious new life that was a part of her. Mom had experience caring for young children from her days in foster care, but nothing in her life had taught her you could love like this. She would protect Louise for the rest of her life.

On the morning Mom was to be discharged from the hospital, she fed Louise and reluctantly surrendered her to the nurses. They would prepare Louise for discharge while Mom dressed and packed. The nurses took Louise to dress her in the tiny white booties, bonnet, and sweater set Mom had crocheted during her pregnancy.

A soft knock on Mom's door announced a visitor. Looking up, she watched the doctor let himself into the room. Mom's nervous system began to sound the alarm the minute he walked in the door. *There is that which we can see and that which we cannot see.* Mom's finely tuned trauma radar was on high alert. He looked at her and said, "I think you should sit down." Mom was always careful with her recall here. She said he looked at her and spoke, "I don't know how to tell you this, so I am just going to say it. Your beautiful baby is dead." Mom passed out.

She spent several more days in the hospital, too distraught to imagine going on without Louise. I wonder now if this was actually the beginning of

Chapter Ten: Roses

Mom's heart breaking. I have in my possession the old worn and yellowed baby book Mom had started for Louise. I don't ever remember seeing this before. Mom and I came across it when we were clearing her belongings in preparation for her death. Not one to keep sentimental objects, I surprised myself by asking Mom if I could have it. I still have it. Mom's seventeen-year-old hand had carefully filled in the prompts. She recorded Louise's birth weight and height. The space for weight and height upon discharge is still blank.

Each page is adorned with cutouts of yellow chicks or storks or Gerber-looking babies in matching bonnets and dresses that Mom had cut from magazines. The pamphlet from the hospital that all new mothers received entitled "How to Care for Your Baby" is there. In the section for cards, there are five old-fashioned, faded cards with simple greetings that welcome your new baby. Mom's circle was small. She had recorded the gifts she had received for Louise: five nightshirts, three blankets, one sweater set, twelve diapers. On the page where you record your baby's health record, Mom had noted an upset stomach that did not last long on day two of Louise's life. The page entitled "Family Tree" was blank on my mother's side other than Mom and only partially filled in on my father's side.

As I write this, I realize that Mom never kept another baby book after Louise despite having five more children. The cause of Louise's death was never fully identified. Does it qualify as Sudden Infant Death Syndrome when the child is only five days old? There was no reason to suspect anything like this might happen. She was born a beautiful healthy baby girl—*maybe too beautiful for this world?* When they brought Mom her baby so she might say goodbye, Louise was dressed in her white going-home outfit. The thing Mom remembers vividly and describes whenever she tells this story is the small trickle of blood that ran out of one of Louise's tiny nostrils and trickled down her cheek. At this point in the telling, she would often break down and ask me, "Why, Theresa? Why couldn't they have wiped that blood away?" As I write these words, my eyes are filled with water.

I feel the remnants of the trauma Mom experienced. Like osmosis, this trauma has permeated all of her children's cells with each telling of the

Chapter Ten: Roses

story. Even though we didn't know her, Louise is part of our family and the loss affected all of our lives. Mom mourned Louise for the rest of her life. At the funeral, the tiny casket was covered with yellow roses. In the baby book is a dried and faded red rose that my father brought to Mom upon learning of Louise's death. This is why there are no roses in Mom's garden. There have never been any roses in Mom's gardens. We grew up knowing never to give Mom roses for any occasion, especially yellow roses.

We have arrived in Milton. The sun is shining and all of our stomachs are growling. This is not the sleepy little town we grew up in. Milton has been incorporated into the sprawling area of Mississauga and become an extension of Toronto. Despite this urban growth, we are able to find some of the important landmarks from our youth. We stopped at a deli and ordered sandwiches and chips. We had a picnic in Victoria Park, the park we played in as children. We drove up the Niagara Escarpment to Rattlesnake Point. This was a favorite landing spot for us as young children. We were all hungry for memories to sustain us through the grief already silently breaking our hearts.

After Louise, Mom prayed that she would get pregnant again. On October 15, just days after returning home from the hospital, while studying Nona's liturgical calendar, she realized that it was the feast day of Saint Teresa of Avila. Mom began to pray to Saint Teresa daily. She prayed for a healthy baby, for another chance to be a mother. She promised Saint Teresa that if she could have a healthy baby, she would name all of her daughters in honor of her. I was born a little over a year later on October 21, 1959. I was christened Theresa after a promise made by Mom to Saint Teresa. My middle name is Eloise in honor of my sister Louise. Both of my sisters bear the name Teresa as their middle names. Mom kept her promise.

Mom was allowed to keep me with her in the hospital. She had cried hysterically when she woke and I was gone. The distraught nurses contacted the doctor, and he instructed them to bring me to Mom no matter the time of day or night when she asked. He understood her fear after having lost Louise. Mom's third child, my middle sister, arrived on November 23, 1960. Her fourth child, my youngest sister, was born March 14, 1962. My brother was born June 1, 1965.

Chapter Ten: Roses

With each pregnancy Mom was having more severe and unrelenting morning sickness and difficult deliveries. The doctor had implored her to begin using birth control pills, and with each child Mom would talk with the priest. Despite the health risks to Mom and her babies, the answer from the priest was always no. Remember, Mom was invested in becoming not only a good Catholic, but a *great* Catholic. Mom's last baby was born in the summer of 1966. Maria was the sixth child she carried to term over a period of eight years.

Mom sensed from the very beginning that there was something wrong and Maria would not live. The same doctor had delivered all of us and scolded Mom for saying such things. He told her she was just afraid because of what had happened with Louise. He insisted Maria was fine, but Mom knew Maria was not fine. During her entire pregnancy she did not prepare the nursery or make any arrangements for bringing this child home. On the day that Maria was born, Mom struggled for hours to push her out. She was in the breech position. Her feet were where her head should have been in the birth canal. Finally, the doctor put Mom under anesthesia while they worked to deliver Maria.

Mom has little memory of this delivery. What she does remember is beginning to wake from the anesthesia in an empty room. In the silence, she turned her head toward the entrance to the room, and there in the doorway she saw a vision of Mother Mary holding a baby. Mom knew it was her baby. Before she left the hospital after Maria's birth, she had a tubal ligation. She was finished delivering babies. I was seven years old when Maria was born. I don't have any clear memories of that time other than all of us children being sent to stay with aunts and friends for several weeks just before and following Maria's birth. Mom went to a convent and sequestered herself so she could grieve and pray and rest. I don't remember that we ever talked about Maria as a family. *Mom did the remembering for all of us.*

We park the car by the cemetery and find the two small grave markers slightly overgrown with grass and weeds showing us where our sisters are buried. Where Mom's other daughters are buried. My sisters and I stood in silence for a long while with Mom and silently held her up with our love while she made one last visit to her oldest daughter Louise and her youngest daughter Maria. If they were alive today, Louise

Chapter Ten: Roses

would have just turned sixty-two and Maria would be fifty-three. If it was possible, I prayed Mom would be reunited with her daughters on November 15.

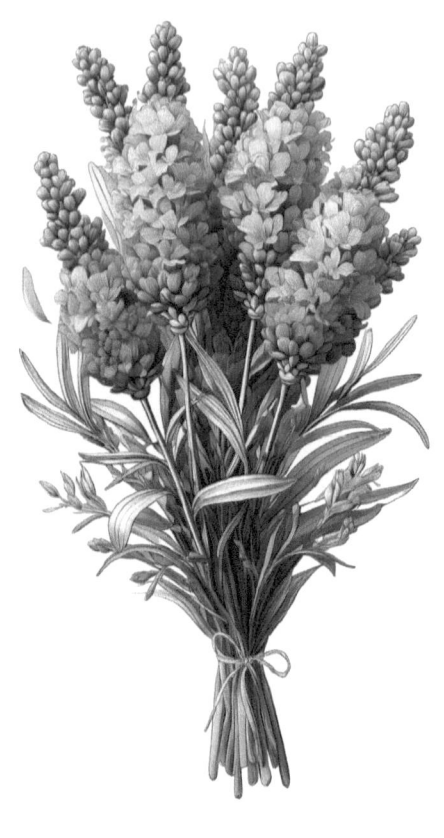

Lavandula

Common Name – Lavender

*Lavender plants can grow as tall as two feet and as wide
as three feet. Mom has collected the flowers that shoot up
on the bare rectangular spiked stems for two summers.
She has filled three sachets with the flowers.
One for each of her daughters.*

Chapter Eleven

Lavender

Journal entry November 1, 2020. *As I crawled into bed tonight, I wished the days would not spin quite so fast... but today Mom looked so exhausted, so ready. She told me she was worried that her grandchildren would not understand. I listened. I reminded her that they all have mothers, and those mothers are her daughters. That we would all be here to support our children and listen to them as they grieved the loss of their Grams. Fourteen days until November 15.*

I can't walk through Mom's garden or any garden without pausing to let my hands caress the lavender plants. I let my hands become my eyes as they feel the rough woody texture just below the surface that is covered with thousands of soft, slender leaves whose shape is that of pine needles. The touch of my hands releases a scent that is aromatic and sweet and carries hints of pine and the forest. Like a healing balm, the familiar fragrance envelops me. I cover my face with my hands and breathe in the calm carried on these tiny invisible molecular atomizers.

Lavender plants have leaves, stems, and flowers that are covered in trichomes or tiny hairs. Embedded amongst these hairs are glands that produce the aromatic oil we associate with lavender. Lavender oil has been studied for its calming and relaxing effects. It is used to reduce anxiety and foster relaxation. I let my attention drop into the soles of my feet and connect deeply with the earth. Right now, I am living more in my mind and my heart. Thoughts and feelings seem to outweigh physical sensations. Whenever we are absorbed in something intensely, unless that intensity is of a physical origin, we tend to forget about our body. Our nervous system normalizes this heightened way of being and our muscles never completely release to rest, even when we sleep. Like anything we practice long enough, this way of being becomes a habit. Tension becomes a habit. *Tension feels like rest.*

Prolonging this invitation to drop back into my body, I kick my Birkenstocks off so I can wiggle my

Chapter Eleven: Lavender

toes in the dirt. Silently, I give thanks for these late October days that carry the warmth of mid-September. It has snowed in the past on my birthday, and here I am with bare feet! Mom has concrete stepping-stones in her garden that have been molded using giant rhubarb leaves. They have become hidden under four years of earth and mulch and appear like buried treasures as I work in different sections of the garden. The veins molded in the stones are prominent and draw an intricate map from the base of the leaf to the apex or tip.

Nature is art. I step carefully onto the first steppingstone and pause. We are past the halfway point on our journey with Mom. Destination unknown. Some days it feels like we forgot the map and are completely lost. Other days feel like we are right on course. When I arrived here in mid-August, ninety days felt like enough time. Now it is November 1 and I want the pages of the calendar to start turning in reverse. My right foot lands carefully on the next steppingstone and I pause, balancing on one leg. A memory that carries so much joy fills my consciousness.

My sisters and I are drawing the squares and numbers for hopscotch using colored chalk. As I close my eyes and let this memory sweep through me, I let my feet land thoughtfully on each concrete rhubarb leaf in Mom's garden. Any hopscotch aficionada knows the secret weapon is finding the right stone that can land precisely on the chosen square without skipping ahead or jumping off to the right or left. We spent hours playing outside as children. Pouring out the door once our chores were completed and showing up in time for dinner, having bicycled and skipped and climbed our way all over town and back.

Each summer Mom would stitch a season pass to the local pool onto our new swimsuits. We would arrive at the Jaycee's pool when the gates opened and leave when the gates closed. Even the mandated rest periods by the lifeguards felt like too much time out of the water. After passing a swimming test, you earned the right to swim in the "big kid's" pool. This was all well and good and definitely a move up the status ladder, but a larger and taller issue presented itself. Who would risk life and limb and be the first to jump off the high diving board? Our youngest sister was usually our test subject when it came to risky ventures, and this is how she became the first one to jump. We figured if she made it out alive, we were golden.

I have a lot of happy memories playing as a child. Mom reminds me that I never walked anywhere. I skipped, I hopped, I ran, I climbed, I cartwheeled, I skated, I rolled; my career as a movement educator started when I was young. As we grew older, Mom started taking us to play bingo with her. Mom loves bingo. Actually, Mom loves gambling. I think of bingo as the sanctioned Catholic form of gambling. My sisters and I have planned a last bingo game for Mom. She is far too weak to go out for bingo, so we will bring bingo to her. It's a surprise for her. We have bought an official bingo cage with the numbered balls. Bingo cards and new bingo daubers. We have enlisted my sister's husband to be the caller. Most of the prizes are scratch tickets, another favorite of Mom's.

I am almost finished putting the garden to rest. Who will tend this garden when Mom is gone? Will they love it and care for it the way Mom has? I cannot create any expectations for this. In fourteen days, Mom will leave her physical body behind. She will leave her garden behind. She will leave her children behind. From that moment on, she will live in my heart. She will live in my memories. She will live in the DNA that migrated from her cells and helped create my cells.

I inspect Mom's lavender for any signs of root rot such as yellowing or browning leaves. I know that lavender is susceptible to root rot as it has happened in my own garden. Most of us tend to water plants too much rather than too little. The soil must drain adequately, and lavender requires six hours of sunlight to really thrive. Mom has a healthy patch of lavender that she has nourished with full sunlight and careful watering.

This is English lavender, which is able to withstand the cooler northern climates. The fragrant leaves are a soft cloudy green in color. The flowers draw in the bees with hues of lavender blue petals. Lavender plants are herbaceous perennials that grow like evergreen shrubs. They can grow as tall as two feet and as wide as three feet. Mom has collected the flowers that shoot up on the bare rectangular spiked stems for two summers. She has filled three sachets with the flowers. One for each of her daughters. I love how Mom has showered us with

Chapter Eleven: Lavender

her love through these thoughtful little acts. She is very aware of how painful this will be for all of us. She has felt the pain of the loss of a mother. While having your mother exit via MAID is a bit overwhelming, losing a mother you never really had carries its own special grief.

I put my tools away and head into the house. I have been painting the kitchen so it will feel clean and light and bright for Mom and for when we put it on the market. Last week, we started actively selling Mom's possessions. She urged us to do it. My sister put several items from the kitchen up on Marketplace and we quickly had a response from a young man. Turns out, Wesley has just moved to town for a new job. He bought everything we had listed. In conversation, my sister learns that he needs almost everything you can think of to set up his new apartment, from linens and towels and sheets to dishes and kitchen essentials to laundry supplies, etc. My sister and I look at each other, and she thinks carefully before she speaks. "Wesley, if you can be patient, maybe for … let's say fourteen more days, we might be able to help you out." This is how most of Mom's household items, including furniture, ended up over at this young man's new apartment. We joked that if we ever get really lonely for Mom, we can head on over to Wesley's and sit at the dining-room table!

Mom is sleeping. I am going to take a nice hot bath and do some journaling. As the steaming water is filling the tub, I add a healthy dose of the lavender oil Mom always has on hand. I will ask my sisters if I can take the rhubarb steppingstones home to my garden.

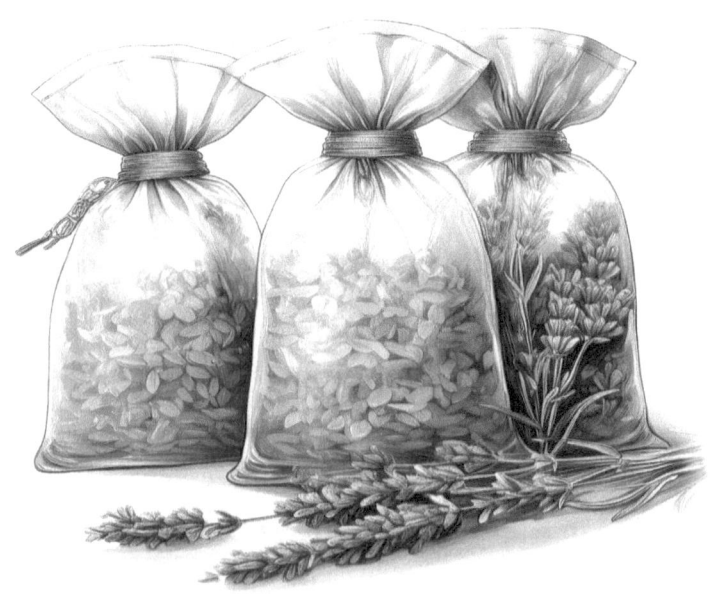

Chapter Eleven: Lavender

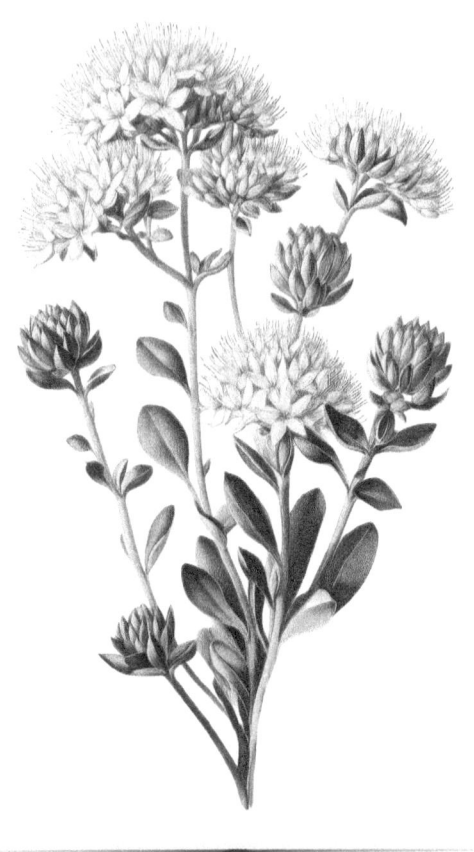

Sedum

Common Name – Stonecrop

Sedums are members of the succulent family. This variety of sedum is named Autumn Joy. Like Autumn Joy, we all wear different crowns during our life. Some we choose and some we inherit. Some we wear for years and others we toss because they no longer fit.

Chapter Twelve

SEDUM

Journal entry November 2, 2020. Have been getting the house ready for sale. Today I felt the depth of the hole that will be left when Mom leaves. The sobs came. I felt the fatigue. I could barely get through teaching my online somatic movement class. I am not going to teach for the rest of November. I went upstairs and found Mom resting in bed. I lay beside her and wrapped my arms and legs around her. I smelled her mother-scent. I felt her mother-love. Thirteen more days until November 15.

The colorful blooms of summer are over, and we have slipped into the season of rest. The garden is almost tucked in for the winter. Most of the plants have been cut back and covered with dry leaves and mulch. My sisters have moved plants from Mom's garden into their own gardens. I have my seeds safely tucked away with planting instructions from

Mom for my return home. Paul's boots now rest in my youngest sister's garden. Next year she will fill those boots with red geraniums.

There is one plant still flowering in the garden. A spectacular fall-blooming sedum. Most of the plants in Mom's garden are deciduous and have dropped all of their leaves. Their flowers have turned to seedpods. The seedpods have dried and the seeds have dropped. Some land in close proximity, while others are carried on autumn winds. Many more seeds have been scattered than will germinate in the spring, *as if nature is hedging her bet.*

Sedums are members of the succulent family. This variety of sedum is named Autumn Joy. *Even Mom's plants can show up as joy.* Succulents store water in their leaves, stems, and roots. This is reflected in their fleshy leaves and stalks. Mom's feet, ankles, and legs are also fleshy right now as they store the fluids her heart and her kidneys are no longer able to circulate effectively. Autumn Joy emerges in the spring like a crowded patch of miniature cabbage plants or Brussels sprouts resting on the dark earth. The serrated edges add even more interest to mint gray-green leaves that are color washed in translucent yellows and contrast the dark green hues of the neighboring plants. The stalks can reach two feet in height and two feet in width as they grow into large dense circles under the direction of their DNA.

I wonder if Mom's siblings struggled with health issues like she has. Our family history is spotty at best. I know I have aunts and uncles and most likely many cousins, but like seeds scattered in the fall, the seeds of my parents' families have landed far from the mother-plant. Sometimes, a seed lands and manages to germinate despite adverse conditions. All living organisms—including plants, animals, and humans—have molecules that determine their instructions for life. In the center of every single cell, DNA carries the blueprint for the development, functioning, growth, and reproduction for all organisms.

When a seed lands in the "barely there" crack in a sidewalk, germinates, and produces a plant, enough of the operating instructions have been met. Maybe not enough to grow a thriving multibranched herbaceous plant that will bear abundant fruit ... but occasionally I have come across just such a plant while walking a city street, happily blooming in the midst of the dust, concrete, and litter of the city. *We are hardwired to survive.*

When we garden, there are times we make the choice for the plant. If a plant grows beyond its intended boundaries, we can simply separate it into two or more clumps destined for a new location or maybe a friend's garden. If volunteers germinate in a location we do not find desirable, they can quickly be pulled out and thrown into the compost pile. The joke is on us when that very same plant shows up in all its glory the following spring growing right out of that very same compost pile! *All it takes is one seed to germinate.*

Mom told me she had pruned her Autumn Joy in the late spring. It was looking a bit leggy as it was being crowded out by other plants. Autumn Joy loves six hours of sunlight each day to thrive. It is suggested that you cut the plant back by half in late spring or early summer. This will delay blooming but produce a stronger, bushier plant with more blooms. The blooms form in an umbel shape. Think umbrella. A flower cluster with stems that are close to equal in length grow from a common center. The tightly closed buds form a flat or slightly curved surface. Pruning and creating space for more sun has given the sedum in Mom's garden optimum conditions to grow toward the full potential of its DNA program.

Chapter Twelve: Sedum

Sedums wear a different crown of florets for every season. In the early summer, they look like a cousin to broccolini, with clusters of buds at the top of their stalks still reflecting sun-washed mint greens. When the buds begin to open into tiny star-shaped petals in late summer, they take on a light pink hue that deepens with time. By late September subtle pink hues have morphed into bright coral-red florets that will transition to a deep rusty red-brown color in late fall. The flowers on Mom's sedum are transitioning from vibrant pink to deep burnt sienna.

Like Autumn Joy, we all wear different crowns during our life. Some we choose and some we inherit. Some we wear for years and others we toss because they no longer fit. This was certainly true of Mom. She worked as a Certified Nursing Assistant in long-term care facilities during our primary school years. She was a caregiver. She was a comforter. As children, my sisters and I spent Sunday afternoons in the nursing home passing out fruit from a basket and singing the old songs from the forties that Mom had taught us.

Mom also had a special way of being with people who were dying. She was never afraid. She could simply stay present for the process. No one died alone on Mom's shifts. When my parents purchased their farm, she learned how to help birth horses, how to groom them and care for them after a race. She learned how to raise chickens, milk a cow, and drive a tractor. When money was tight, she worked in a factory that manufactured aluminum windows.

My father left when Mom was just forty-six. They had lived together slightly shy of thirty years. Even though my sisters and I saw this as liberation for her, for Mom it was another loss that would take her some time to recover from. In time, she began to leave behind the fantasy that someone else could be responsible for her happiness and learned to cultivate happiness on her own.

At the age of fifty, Mom decided to become a magician and a clown. She wanted to take her joy to the children and adults in hospitals. Years ago, when I was sorting through my own growing pains, I remember reading somewhere that it is not possible to skip a developmental stage of growth. Here was Mom doing all the playing she had missed as a child in the guise of a clown. Her name was *Dandeelion,* and children and adults alike loved her.

Chapter Twelve: Sedum

She went to Clown College in Florida. She purchased oversized purple clown shoes with pink daisies for closures that complemented the purple plaids she had sewn into ruffled skirts and petticoats. She wore a crown of bouncy yellow curls with a straw hat adorned with a dandelion. She supported her expensive clown habit by sewing elaborate special-order costumes for other clowns. Just like Mom had sewn Barbie clothes for the kids at school when she was a young girl, she was harnessing all of her skills and showing up as joy.

Mom had a knack for magic tricks and practiced like a young lawyer preparing for the bar exam. She clowned in parades, at private birthday parties, company events, and town festivals. She got around. Her car had giant magnetic polka dots that announced Dandeelion was in the room. Clowning can be an expensive proposition. When Mom needed extra money for a new trick to add to her bag, she would dress up as Dandeelion and head out to the local parks for some good old-fashioned busking. *She was both afraid and fearless at the same time.* Her most sought-after talent as a clown was face painting. She was an artist, and this translated into elaborate designs carefully painted onto the faces of eager children who waited in line to meet Dandeelion.

There is a magnolia tree in Mom's garden. The branches are bare now, and the blooms long gone. One of the world's oldest flowering trees, magnolia tree fossils reveal they were alive over *one hundred million years ago*. They even predated bees, and so they evolved to be pollinated by beetles that are attracted to their scent. *Jim-dad* bought this flowering deciduous tree for Mom. Each season when the first bud begins to unfurl, Mom thanks Jim. She's sure it is a gift from her beloved. They were soul partners who met several years after Mom's divorce. He was a gentle giant who needed Mom as much as she needed him. He appeared when Mom had lost faith in most humans, and they had twenty-five years together. Not a conventional marriage, but on terms that worked for both of them. I know she is hoping they will somehow be reunited on her birthday this year. I hope so.

Despite my sixty years of living the changing of the seasons, there is always a moment when I am jolted into the realization that the season *has actually changed*. It seems like a slow transformation

Chapter Twelve: Sedum

until it is not. The summer solstice marks the beginning of summer and occurs on June twentieth or twenty-first in the Northern Hemisphere where I live. The Latin word for *solstice* means *the sun stands.* This is the longest day of the year, averaging fifteen to sixteen hours of daylight; it's a booster shot that charges all of life after the dark days of winter.

Between winter and summer comes *spring.* Each year the first warmish sunny day I can venture outside without boots and a winter jacket my senses come alive and I feel liberated. My skin drinks in the sun and my nostrils draw in the scents that have been buried in the frozen turf of the winter months. The first day of spring is called the *vernal equinox* and happens on March nineteenth, twentieth, or twenty-first. The earth's orbit and axis line up, and in this position, the earth's axis is not tilted toward or away from the sun. Northern and Southern Hemispheres experience an equal amount of light and dark. The Latin words that make up *equinox* mean *equal night.*

We have already passed the *autumnal equinox,* which occurred on September twenty-third. All of the seasons come and go in relation to the earth's tilt and rotation around the sun. Maybe the element of surprise comes because we are gaining or losing daylight in a minute or minutes every day during the calendar year. *Season creep* is the slow process (measured in decades) of the gradual shifting of the timing of the seasons. Where I live, we are experiencing an earlier spring and a later fall. Mom has lived eighty years of changing seasons in her body. She has shown up for each season the best that she was able. Some of her life has been lived in the darkness and some in the light—and then there are all the moments in-between. *There is that which we can see and that which we cannot see.* Even perennials have a life span.

I will leave the sedum as it stands. The dried flowers will retain their color and contain the seeds that will provide another source of food for winter birds.

Chapter Twelve: Sedum

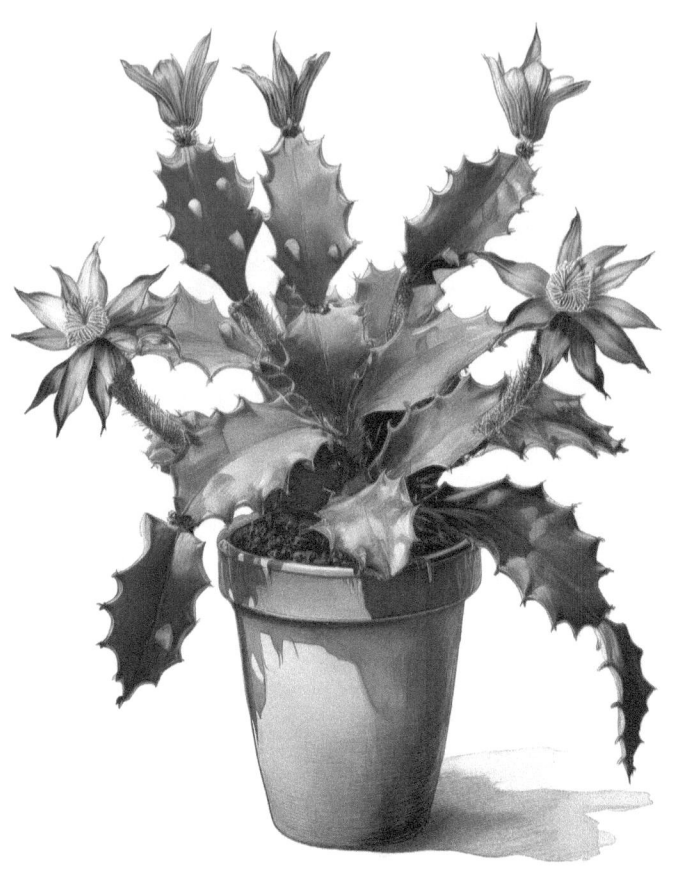

Schlumbergera
Common Name – Christmas Cactus

This Christmas Cactus is the only plant that lives inside Mom's house. It has inhabited Mom's home long enough to have become part of her story. She is going to split the cactus for us so we can each take a piece home.

Chapter Thirteen

CHRISTMAS CACTUS

Journal entry November 3, 2020. Sitting in the living room with Mom and my sisters. The house has been transformed and feels light and bright and spacious. Mom loves it. She is so eager to clear her space. No attachments to stuff. We have twelve days left to celebrate with Mom before we lift her to the light. Twelve more days until November 15.

My focus has shifted from the garden. With everything neat and tidy and tucked in for the winter, the new owners will inherit the fruits of Mom's vision for this tiny speck of earth. They may change it, or they may fall under invisible spells cast by the beautiful flora. Either way must be fine. Concrete rhubarb steppingstones now take up space in my car. They will lay a new path in my own garden as literal foundations for shaky steps into my first year without Mom.

Whoever inhabits this house after Mom will inherit the home that has been the backdrop for four years of my family's history. *This bland, tiny square house on a slightly run-down street, in a more than slightly run-down city.* Mom was right, this house has provided a perfect place for healing. Not too big and not too small. Close to the hospital and a pharmacy that delivers. Close to both of my sisters and my brother Paul while he was alive. Neighbors we might never have chosen who have now become friends. Friends who have loved Mom and loved Mom's garden. Mom's beautiful, bountiful, glorious garden. *Mom's last earthly home.* Who knows what is to come, but I imagine she will be unencumbered by four walls and a foundation.

My sisters and I have been using all the skills we have learned from Mom over the years. Cleaning every nook and cranny and gradually applying a fresh coat of paint to each of the rooms has brightened things up. I keep looking to Mom for signs that she wants us to slow down or stop the process of preparing the house for sale, but she is reveling in

Chapter Thirteen: Christmas Cactus

the progress. I can't stop my heart from digging for buried treasures to bring home these days. *I don't really need another stainless slotted kitchen spoon, but I don't have any stainless slotted kitchen spoons that Mom has used countless times over the years as she stirred her pasta sauce.*

The realtor is coming this week. A friend of my sisters since childhood. She is aware of the plans. Mom wants to set the price, approve the photos, and in general make sure all the i's are dotted and the t's are crossed. This will be the twelfth house Mom has owned during her adult life. I think we all love moving. It's part of our DNA. Carried down in our genes. My Irish maternal grandparents and my Italian paternal grandparents all crossed the sea to immigrate to Canada, while we traversed southwestern Ontario.

Mom has an octagonal side table made of wood that has darkened with age. The patina is a warm walnut. Heavily carved leaves and vines wind their way up and down five pairs of legs and circle the round perimeter. She does not have sentimental pieces of furniture. Collecting treasures from her ancestors was never an option. This table is different. A Mother's Day gift from her teenage daughters. Wooden validation that she has been a good mother. For over forty years this table has moved from house to house to house with Mom. Now it will reside in my sister's home. I secretly pine for it, but I recognize this as a false sense of security that relies on me surrounding myself with *Mom stuff.* As if this will blunt the sensation of missing her when she is gone.

Mom's Christmas cactus lives in the center of this vine-covered table. This is the only plant that lives *inside* Mom's house. This cactus has inhabited Mom's home long enough to have become part of her story. She is going to split the cactus for us so we can each take a piece home. Round stone pots the color of dark jade will hold our treasures. Holes in the bottom of the pots will drain the excess moisture that could lead to disease and root rot. Cactus soil mix amended specifically for succulents will feed and anchor the plant's roots in the soil. *Invisible golden threads will anchor the daughters to the mother.*

Christmas cacti are part of the succulent family. The leaves show me they are designed to store water by their waxy coating, called the cuticle. Transpiration occurs when a plant releases water

Chapter Thirteen: Christmas Cactus

vapor through its leaves. Think of this as an exhalation. The cuticle helps to slow the process of transpiration. Stomata, the minuscule pores covering the surface of the waxy leaves, will facilitate the release of water vapor. Plants lose up to ninety-nine percent of their water via transpiration. Most plants open their stomata during the day. Christmas cacti open theirs only at night, which helps slow the process of water evaporation even further.

Looking at Mom's Christmas cactus reminds me that she will not be here for Christmas. Mom won't mind. Christmas has never been one of her favorite holidays. When Mom was a child, Christmas was a grim reminder of everything she didn't have. Mom's desire to grow her happy family outweighed her dislike for Christmas. A rebound effect would take place every year as she threw herself into every Christmas tradition known to Catholics.

Weeks before December twenty-fifth, Mom's fruitcake would appear in the dank basement where candied cherries and nut meats slowly absorbed the brandy that would create the deep, rich flavor. Mincemeat pies, spritz and sugar cookies, peanut butter blossoms, almond snowballs, coconut macaroons, shortbread, peanut brittle, toffee, and other treats would appear in every shape and size and begin to fill the freezer. I am sure my sisters and I sampled these goodies as soon as we figured out what was going on. Eventually, the cookies and cakes and candies would fill silver holiday trays bursting with color and texture and the fruits of Mom's hands to be shared with family, friends, and neighbors. A fresh short-needled pine tree decorated with ornaments, lights, and tinsel marked the resting place for the holy manger and its occupants. An angel graced the top with just enough sparkle to convince young children that magic was real.

Each year families were asked to donate gingerbread houses to our school, Saint Michael's Elementary. The annual Christmas raffle was an important fund-raiser. Mom would bake the gingerbread from scratch. Her engineering mind helped her construct the elaborate walls and roof lines of the gingerbread house. Her deft hands squeezed frosting from aluminum-tipped pastry bags brought out once each year for this special occasion. Icing piped and swirled over and around the gingerbread, while doubling as mortar to hold the house together.

Chapter Thirteen: Christmas Cactus

Candy in various shapes and colors masqueraded as shingles, windows, doors, and siding. My sisters and I were mesmerized by Mom's creations. She was an artist. These were no ordinary gingerbread houses. They were the most sought-after gingerbread houses at the annual school raffle.

Journal entry November 5, 2020. Mom was talking a lot in her sleep last night. There was a moment when it felt like restlessness and I wondered if I should wake her. I decided not to. This morning, I helped her with her shower. She rested her forehead on my chest while I dried her hair and rubbed her favorite lotion into her fragile skin. Mom was still taking independent baths when I arrived August 12. Since then, she has gone from independent bathing to bathing only when someone else is in the house, and later to being bathed. Mom has always loved her baths. Steamy hot bubbly water.

The strength to carry out this basic activity of daily living is no longer available. She can't get up or down to take a bath. A white plastic shower chair inhabits the back half of Mom's tub. My sisters and I now bathe her. It takes effort to help her onto and off of the shower chair. The whole thing exhausts her. The progression is right. The physical events are escalating. Mom seems to be shedding cells faster and faster. Her naps are frequent, but she is still light and bright. Nine more days until November 15.

The weather is finally beginning to reflect late fall. My sisters and I are sitting outside on the porch in front of Mom like we did when we were young. Like three newly hatched chicks, we wait with our mouths wide open for any morsel she may throw our way. Mom is getting ready to leave the nest. Her chicks have returned home to help her with the leaving. She is dividing her Christmas cactus.

Mom insisted on dividing the plant with her own hands. We had planned to do this yesterday, but she was too tired. With the serrated bread knife from the kitchen that has not yet found its way over to Wesley's apartment, Mom is carefully dividing the cactus into three equal clumps. It feels like a ceremony. We are listening to her instructions intently, like we did as young children when she would tell us a story or teach us a song.

"OK, girls, six weeks before you want the plant to bloom, water it really well and place it in a dark,

Chapter Thirteen: Christmas Cactus

cool closet. It needs at least twelve hours of darkness every day. Water it just enough to keep the soil barely moist. Once you see the buds, you can bring it back out into a bright location and water it normally."

We are so aware of each other's presence right now that words often feel redundant. This house is special to Mom because she *owns* this house. She has a small mortgage that will easily be covered by the sale. Any other profits will be split between her three daughters. Mom has asked us to call this *our house* from now on. She wants to hear us take ownership of the house. Her gift to us. Mom never had any of this while growing up. She has broken the cycles of poverty and abandonment that marked much of her early years.

She has a forty-thousand-dollar term life insurance policy that she has been paying on for thirty years. The last few years, my sister and I have covered it as Mom was adamant about not letting it lapse, and her fixed income was proving inadequate. She has paid way more than forty thousand dollars in small monthly increments over the years, but that is not important to her. Each payment has been an investment and a testament to her love for her children. An added bonus is the current housing market. It has exploded in the four years since Mom bought her home.

The weather has turned colder, and we have tucked Mom into her chair with a steaming cup of tea. My sisters and I are thrilled with our new plants. They sit side by side on the table waiting to be carried to their respective homes.

She sits in her chair knitting with a look of contentment. She has something to leave her daughters. A tangible expression of her love.

Part Three

WINTER'S APPROACH

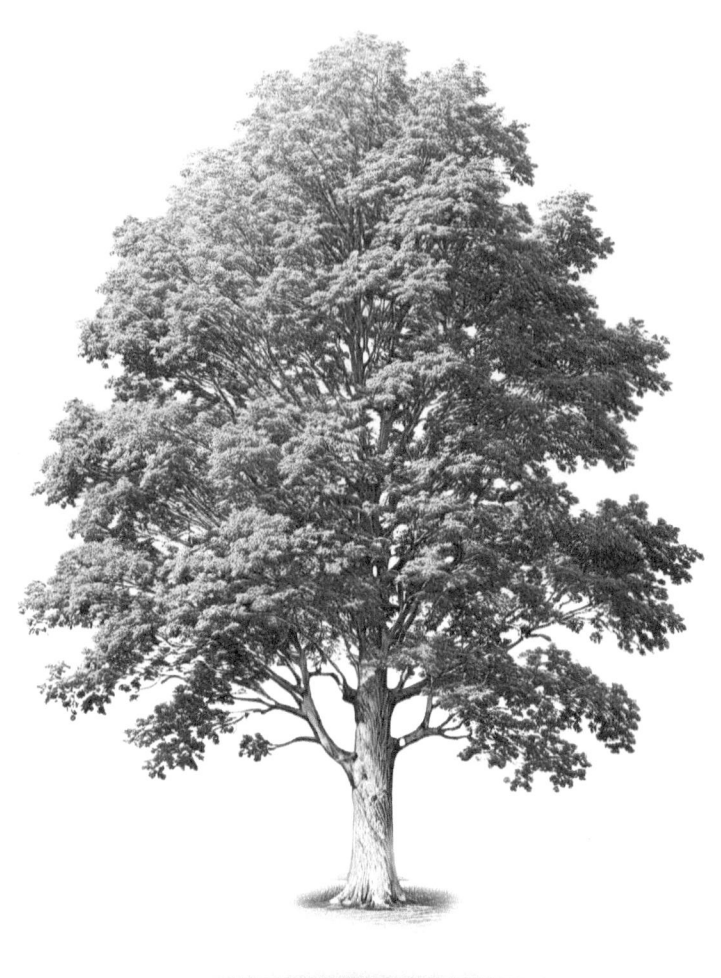

Acer saccharum
Common Name – Sugar Maple Tree
Maple trees come in all shapes and sizes and colors. Each tree with a certain percentage of shared DNA and each tree with individuated DNA. Like families.

Chapter Fourteen

Sugar Maple Tree

Journal entry November 8, 2020. *I am going through Mom's jewelry box with her tonight. She is giving the box to my daughter. The jewelry is bringing back memories of Mom when she loved to wear funky jewelry and many different kinds. Some I recognize because I gave them to her. There are pieces I have never seen Mom wear. This is bringing me close to the sense of loss I will feel when Mom leaves her body next Sunday.*

NO! But YES! Be free, Mom, be free. It is time. It is only for selfish reasons that I would wish it any different. I will welcome the deep visceral sense of loss and sorrow I will feel when you depart. I will recognize it as reflecting the importance of our relationship. I chose you to be my mother. You have been one of the greatest influences in my life. You have been a constant, really, the most constant. It is my honor to serve you now in the last days of your life. Seven more days until November 15.

Mom has a gigantic maple tree that overhangs her back deck. It is actually in the neighbor's yard, but they share it. It is packed with shimmering yellow leaves tinted with oranges and reds whose colors turn iridescent when they glisten in the sun. It's a sugar maple, but honestly, it mostly looks like any of the hundreds of maple trees that dot this small city. Like maple trees, my sisters and I *mostly* look like each other these days. We are 57, 58, and 61 years old now. We bring our wisdom and our wounds. We are trying to be tender with each other, and mostly we are, but there are moments we spill all over each other like the sap that runs from these hardwood trees in the early spring. The sensations we are feeling erupt and stick to everything. It's always over something completely insignificant because those are the things it is safe to be angry at, or afraid of, or sad for. Usually, we are quick to recover. We are united by a greater single-mindedness right now.

Maple trees come in all shapes and sizes and colors. Each tree with a certain percentage of shared DNA and each tree with individuated DNA. Like families. This tree has only just begun to drop its leaves

CHAPTER FOURTEEN: SUGAR MAPLE TREE

with the warm autumn weather we have been experiencing. I choose to believe it has held on as a blazing spectacle of nature's wonder for Mom's last days. They are connected, Mom and this tree. One of her favorite photos is of my brother Paul pushing me on the tire swing that hangs from a gnarled old branch.

My younger sister has several ancient maple trees in her parklike back yard. I was over there this morning helping her finish up her gardens for the fall. At one point she stopped raking and fixed her gaze on me. "Theresa, do you realize that at this time next week Mom will be gone? ... I can't imagine how I will live without her. I don't know how I will get through next Sunday." I can feel her confusion. Her sincere lack of comprehension for what we are doing. I say *we* because it feels like *we*. This moment is asking for all of Mom's daughters to show up. We know she is ready because of the way she is showing up. The honeymoon period is over. We are down to the wire.

My sister isn't crying. She isn't falling apart. She is asking me how we show up for something we have absolutely no frame of reference for. As each day brings us closer to November 15, the permanence of Mom's choice is becoming more and more real. Now, seven days before Mom is to die, everything feels too real. No bingo game is going to distract us from this moment. I met my middle sister on my way out the door this morning. She came to hang with Mom while I help my younger sister in her garden. We stopped outside and looked at each other. Collapsing into each other's arms, we shared a powerful moment disguised as a hug. In fact, we were filling each other with our shared experience, our love for Mom, our love for each other, the fortitude that Mom has nurtured in all of us by example.

We are on a journey that seems completely and utterly unfathomable. In seven days, the nurse will come to Mom's house at ten in the morning. She will insert an IV catheter into Mom's vein and leave. Shortly before eleven, the doctor will show up and we will lay down in bed with Mom while he administers the medications that will stop Mom's breathing and send her on her way. I can't bring myself to say *kill her.* Looking back at my sister, I feel completely inept *and* responsible as her older sibling to ease her heart and mind. "You'll do it. We'll all do it. We'll just keep breathing and putting one foot in front of the other like we've done for this whole experience.

Chapter Fourteen: Sugar Maple Tree

We will continue to show up for Mom. We will keep our shit together for Mom. We can do this. You can do this."

Sugar maples are considered flowering plants. They are in the soapberry family under the umbrella Sapindaceae. Their scientific name is *Acer saccharum*. I don't know why this is a surprise to me. Of course, trees are plants. Really big woody plants. Maple trees can reach heights of one-hundred-forty feet and grow forty to fifty feet wide. The maple overhanging Mom's deck is almost a perfect oval, which is typical of their growth pattern.

Each spring Mom complained about the mess this tree made as yellow-green long-stalked clusters of eight to fourteen floppy flowers called panicles would blanket her deck. These maple tree flowers without petals would collude with the wind and scatter themselves without regard for the space around them. When this massive tree with its five-lobed palmate leaves provided shade and a cool interlude in the middle of a hot summer day, Mom would forget all about the mess this tree made in the spring. Palmate leaves resemble an open hand. Their five lobes radiate from a single point and mimic our five fingers. Whenever I am in Mom's kitchen, this tree lures me in with its beauty. *Thousands of hands masquerading as leaves are energetically holding us up with quiet strength.*

There are fleshy fruits like apples and peaches, and there are dry fruits. A samara is a dry fruit that is indehiscent, meaning it does not split open to release the seeds when ripe. Samaras take the shape of wings and can be single or double. Our childhood name for samaras was helicopters or keys. With paper-like wings mimicking helicopters, they would take flight from the massive maple trees that lined the streets of our neighborhood. These winged seeds let the autumn winds guide them to an arbitrary landing place. A potential place to support the DNA program of the seed and germinate a new plant, or a place to decompose. *It could go either way.*

Nature teaches us in metaphors when we pay attention. Mom's story is such an important story to me and to my sisters, and it is certainly important to Mom. But Mom's story is really no different from my story or my daughter's story or your own story. Like samaras taking flight in the fall, any one of us can find ourselves free-falling as we navigate the

Chapter Fourteen: Sugar Maple Tree

winds of change around us. If you live long enough, you eventually reach a moment that confounds you. A moment that you struggle to find a frame of reference for. *This is where my sisters and I find ourselves seven days before Mom is to leave.*

> **Journal entry November 9, 2020.** *Woke with a keen awareness that this is the first day of our final week with Mom in her body. A tearful morning. Looking into Mom's hazel-gray eyes, they are bright and distant. My tears came frequently all morning. The feelings associated with the tears: joy that Mom will be free soon, sweet sadness that there are days left to physically hug and hold Mom, gratitude that I am here now. Six more days until November 15.*

Mom is expecting a visit today from my brother's adult son. He arrives carrying two boxes wrapped in birthday-themed paper, and my breath catches when I realize he has come to celebrate Mom's birthday. He is the only grandchild who does not know that Mom is ending her life on Sunday with MAID. Her eightieth birthday. Mom and I have talked about this. Mom's still-wounded heart over my brother's death has been superimposed on her grandson's heart. This is what we do when we have been repeatedly traumatized. We feel the world through our traumatized hearts. Mom is sure he is too tender to understand.

He is also excited to introduce us to his own son—Mom's sixth great-grandchild. After hearing my great-nephew loves "large trucks," I have procured just such a truck appropriate for a three-year-old. He is currently pushing a large yellow dump truck with big black nubby tires around Mom's living room. My brother's son is Mom's ninth grandchild. We have almost finished knitting the scarves. *Yes, we are all still knitting.* After Mom wraps him and his son into their scarves, she will have wrapped all of her grandchildren and all of her great-grandchildren into countless knit and purl stitches that form an invisible bond made visible by the soft yarn. *There is that which we can see and that which we cannot see…*

There are conditions that stress sugar maples and convince them that death is imminent. A drought the previous year, unusually warm winters that diminish the growth of new shoots, and fungal infections are three such conditions. If the tree thinks it is going to

Chapter Fourteen: Sugar Maple Tree

die, it will put out many more samaras or seeds than usual in a *final attempt to survive*. More samaras mean more seeds and a greater chance of germination, ensuring the continuation of the species.

A memory surfaces of my sisters and me among the roots of an ancient maple tree in Pinafore Park. We loved to climb those roots. They wear a covering of dark gray, almost black furrowed and grooved bark. Early in a maple's life the bark is smooth and light gray. Its fissures are laid down over the years like the wrinkles that appear around our mouths and eyes with age. Life lays down grooves with each moment lived. These roots make perfect benches for our eight-, ten-, and eleven-year-old bodies. Our knees are bent. Our hands are folded neatly on our laps. Dressed in matching cardigans that Mom has hand-knit, each cardigan is identical except for color. Mine is red, my middle sister's is a soft green, and our youngest sister's is Mom's favorite yellow. I have seen the picture hundreds of times. My brother is also in this picture. His eyes are bright. He is holding a dandelion. *His aura has yet to dim.*

My brother's son has no idea this will be the last time he will see his Grams. My heart is quietly aching for him. He so clearly loves her and is happy to be here. A musician, he is telling us about his current project. He exudes an innocent naivete despite his chaotic upbringing. I pray that if he finds out how Mom left, his heart will not form a scar or burl marking a permanent injury. He has known too much loss in his young life already. He is anxious to be "a good father" for his own young son, but this grandson is still young. Barely an adult. *A sugar maple is a minimum of thirty years old before it even begins to produce seeds.*

> **Journal entry November 10, 2020.** *Met with the funeral director today. A wonderful person. Exceptional. We laughed in the midst of the mundane yet necessary paperwork. There was a moment when I felt I might throw up. I felt it as a real physical somatic sensation. Noted. It's all good. Five more days until November 15.*

Unlike sugar maple samaras, Mom does not want to be buried in the ground. She wants to be cremated. We have made the arrangements. We will call

Chapter Fourteen: Sugar Maple Tree

the funeral director when we are ready to have Mom's body picked up. He will back into the driveway in his everyday minivan and not a hearse. He will come in the back door. No stretcher or rolling cart. He will carry Mom out wrapped in her own blanket with as little fanfare as possible.

Mom's body will spend the night in the funeral home. She wants us to see her body in the morning and watch as they transfer her body into the vehicle that will take her to the crematorium. She wants us to witness her body being transferred into the crematorium chamber. She wants us to push the button that begins the process of cremation with our own hands. Too much social media has convinced Mom that funeral directors try to save money by cremating multiple bodies at once. Even exceptional funeral directors. We all agree that we can do this.

Mom is exhausted when we return from making the funeral arrangements. We tuck her into bed, where she quickly falls asleep. My sisters have left to run some errands. I am in the kitchen doing the dishes and cleaning up. It is another warm sunny day. Warm enough for me to open the back door to Mom's deck so fresh air can fill the room. The sugar maple has finally acknowledged late fall and is dropping golden leaves onto Mom's deck. A slight breeze is playing with the leaves, and several scatter into the kitchen. Smiling, I use Mom's straw broom to sweep them back outside—only to have even more leaves find their way onto the kitchen floor.

This gives me an idea, and I start sweeping the leaves *into* the kitchen. I fill the kitchen and let the leaves find their way into the living room and into the hallway. When Mom wakes, I will transform her home into a forest floor. I can't wait for her to see it. The leaves release organic compounds and other molecules that fill the house with the familiar earthy scent of fall. When Mom wakes, she steps into a five-inch-deep blanket of leaves and looks at me with wide eyes that I can't quite read. "I've filled our house with nature, Mom!" I exclaim.

Why do I feel thirteen again? A long-ago story surfaces. My parents had standardbred horses on their farm. They had a half-mile racetrack for training the horses. One of our frequent jobs was to go out and pick any stones off the track that might cause a horse to trip or throw a shoe. We hated this chore. We were sure working on the chain gang would have been an

Chapter Fourteen: Sugar Maple Tree

easier alternative. One night when my parents were at the races, I gathered my sisters, and we took up arms in the form of rakes and shovels. With a determination fueled by the prospect of never having to collect stones again, we spent hours scraping every bit of loose debris off the track. We couldn't wait to show our parents what a great job we had done. Turns out, we had scraped hundreds of dollars and several years' worth of special topsoil off the track. *Oh boy, this feels like that.*

I help Mom to her chair. Her oxygen hose is picking up leaves along the way. We share a cup of tea surrounded by the sugar maple leaves that have settled into their new environment. Since we have no frame of reference for this journey we are on with Mom, we are writing the script as we live it. Sugar maple leaves are now part of the protocol. I offer to make Mom lunch, but she is not hungry. Her appetite is that of a bird these days. I feel no need to force her to eat. She will eat when she is hungry. Between sips of tea, we are quietly discussing how happy we are with the funeral director we have chosen. Right now, none of us feel the need to fill blank spaces with words. It's enough to be in each other's presence. My sisters will be here soon. Mom wants to watch the movie *Fatima* with us. It is just available for streaming. To visit the site in Portugal where the Virgin Mary appeared to three young children has been on Mom's bucket list. The movie will suffice for now.

Journal entry November 11, 2020. It is evening now. In the past two hours I have felt diminished by the sadness and heartbreak of missing Pete and Stephanie and mixed emotions hearing Mom actually groan with the pain of saying goodbye to two of her grandchildren. Anger, tears, jealousy, love. Why do I feel that I need to apologize for being me right now? But it's already shifting; these sensations are only to be noticed. Information. The sensations are so visceral. Always I feel it most around my heart center. Burning sensations. I am low this moment. I don't feel shiny and bright. I feel like I feel. Four more days until November 15.

Mom has slept most of the day today. She spends more and more time sleeping, and I am convinced a part of her has already started to leave her body. Mom will join the rest of nature in hibernation. She

Chapter Fourteen: Sugar Maple Tree

will drop her body like a dry seedpod. Her seeds have already been distributed and the ancient call to continue the species is complete for this cycle. Her eyes are distant. Her energy is low. It matches mine right now. I wonder if she is willing herself to die. She tells me no, but she is ready. When I start to talk to her about bravery, she cuts me off sharply. "There is nothing brave about this, Theresa. I don't ever want to hear that word again."

We have checked off the "to do" list in preparation for Sunday. We made that important trip to Milton with Mom and found the two small grave markers the size of bricks. Melding into the earth for sixty-one years now, they wear the dappled grays and mossy greens of nature. Like hardy long-lived perennials, they are rooted to the resting place of Louise and Maria. I don't really think the soul or the energy or the spirit of Louise and Maria are in the ground there, but their earthly bodies are. A marker of a moment measured in light years. Mom has carried these two daughters in her heart since they were conceived. *I wonder if she will know them in a different way after Sunday.*

Barely peeking out of the summer lawn, both stones are marked only with the letter "B." It could stand for baby or it could be my father's surname, which started with a B. These are the details that we don't even know we crave. We have three more full days to glean all of the answers. The problem is, *we are not yet aware of many of the questions.*

Mom's house looks better than when she bought it. Most of her furniture is gone. The entire house has been repainted. Little repairs are complete. There is a guy downstairs right now steaming the carpets. The house is almost staged for the sale. The contract with the realtor is signed. The FOR SALE sign will go into the ground by the end of next week. All of Mom's accounts have been closed. We are in possession of her important papers. The funeral preparations are complete.

I have removed the two small glass fruit jars from the side table. They held the water for Mom's watercolors that I would refresh daily. She has not painted for a few weeks now. We are all in possession of our favorite *"Mom paintings."* Her art supplies are packed and will come home with me. I look forward to sharing them with Stephanie as we continue the legacy of the art Mom has inspired all of us to make in our own unique ways.

Chapter Fourteen: Sugar Maple Tree

Mom's garden is all tucked in. Some plants have been moved to my sisters' homes. I have my seeds tucked into my suitcase. We each have an iron trellis to bring to our own gardens. We have split up the gardening tools according to our needs. We have our Christmas cactus plants and instructions for care. We have a copy of Mom's shortbread recipe that she has written out for each of us. We have our sachets of lavender.

Mom has been visited by those she needed to see and has called those she wished to speak with before Sunday. Not to share her plan, but to hear their voices one last time. To express her gratitude for their presence in her life without them really realizing this is what she is doing. We have a list of other folks who will need to be called next week. She has said goodbye and hugged all of her grandchildren mightily. There have been no overt displays of the grief that is to follow, but sweet sacred moments with each child who carries her DNA.

Stephanie and Mom have said their goodbyes over the phone. It breaks my heart that Steph is not able to be here right now, but that is the way it is. She and her bestie Missy have prepared their own ceremony to mark the occasion. Mom has visited her cherished places on the shores of Lake Huron and Lake Erie. The places we frequented growing up. We are all part amphibian, having spent hours and days and weeks soaking in the energy of these Great Lakes.

She has had her last fossil hunt. Her last bingo game. Her last meal from her favorite Chinese restaurant. Rosie is thriving in her new home. I stopped by the vet to inquire just three days ago. Right now, we are all walking around in a state of suspended animation with nothing to distract us from the reality that Mom will be gone in four days. This part feels as coarse as old maple bark. Lined and fissured and rough and gnarly, and as tender as the new shoots that will arrive in the spring. *We told Mom in no uncertain terms that no matter how strong our reaction is at the time she leaves her body, she is not to turn back but to soar toward liberation. She nodded her head yes.*

Journal entry November 12, 2020. Thank you, Mom, sisters, and Stephanie, for holding me up this morning. Three more days until November 15.

✧✧✧

Chapter Fourteen: Sugar Maple Tree

I am praying my rosary these days. At bedtime. I pray for divine intervention to prop me up, to prop all of us up during these last days with Mom alive. I pray for grace. I pray for fortitude. I pray to all of my ancestors to show up for Mom and escort her on this journey. I am familiar with the trio of drugs the doctor will administer on Sunday. I administered them frequently in the cardiac surgical intensive care unit. They are all powerful drugs with rapid onsets that normally require the assistance of a ventilator and close monitoring.

Mom will not have a ventilator. Midazolam is a benzodiazepine that will make Mom sleepy and relieve any anxiety she might be experiencing. I wonder if we should all get a little dose of this one. Propofol is an anesthetic and a sedative. This drug will induce a coma and stop Mom's breathing. Rocuronium is a neuromuscular blocker or paralytic. This drug will paralyze Mom's muscles, including her respiratory muscles. It will also prevent any muscle spasms that are a normal physiological function at the end of life but can cause distress to family members who perceive their loved one as being not all the way dead. We are putting our faith in this protocol. We trust this cocktail of drugs will prevent suffering and give Mom a peaceful and rapid death.

These protocols are not without controversy. In the United States, where the protocols regarding MAID are considered very restrictive by many, individuals must consume the medications on their own. This is often referred to as "assisted suicide." I know that many of us have been touched by a loved one who has died via suicide—including me. MAID is different. We need to reframe the language. Those who have chosen MAID are making an informed decision that gives them control over how and when they will exit their body in light of unremitting suffering that cannot be alleviated.

In the United States, the individual is responsible for taking ninety to one hundred barbiturate pills that have been crushed in water and must be consumed within five minutes. Instructions to mix the barbiturates in sugar water to neutralize the bitter taste don't always work. People have reported throwing up while trying to ingest the bitter liquid. Adding stress to an already stressful situation is the worry that one has not consumed enough barbiturates to *actually* die. Again, it's complicated.

Chapter Fourteen: Sugar Maple Tree

This would be a whole lot more stressful if we had to do it on our own. Mom will receive the medication intravenously, administered by the physician. Mom's veins will take in the elixir like the deep branching roots of the sugar maple and distribute it to all of her cells. Because the doctor is administering the drugs, this is called clinician administered assisted death. A retired physician who has volunteered hundreds of times for the MAID program will administer the cocktail of drugs. We have met him several times. He has kind eyes. He looks at you when he speaks. He is patient and has answered all of our questions countless times. He does this because he believes in the right to die with dignity. *For this physician, his professional responsibility encompasses the entire cycle of life, which includes death.*

Journal entry November 13, 2020. We have one more full day with Mom if she stays through the fifteenth of November at 11:00 a.m. Mostly the days have gone by in an easy organic manner—like days can meander, and all of a sudden it is night. Today has been much lighter for me in my mind and my emotions. To remember that life is not static. We are always moving and shifting. That is all it really takes.

Mom would say, "Love, love, and more love." I bought three bracelets today for myself and my sisters. Moonstone. They are so beautiful and feminine. The moonstone is a symbol of light and hope. Its energy encourages us to embrace new beginnings. Two more days until November 15.

While this feels like an ending, it is also a beginning—especially for Mom. I wish I could peek into her next iteration, but it is not for me to know. I will choose a story that feels right and lets my heart rest in peace over this decision, but I will only learn the truth when I drop my own body. *There is that which we can see and that which we cannot see...*

I hope Mom's next journey will be easier for her than this life has been. She may fly on up to heaven and reunite with her family, her friends, and her children. She may reincarnate quickly into another human being. She may hover as energy in the universe. I really don't know. This is a mystery. Catholics believe the soul separates from the human body. The body decays and the soul goes on to meet God. There are Catholics who believe heaven, purgatory, and

Chapter Fourteen: Sugar Maple Tree

hell are real physical places, and there are those who believe these are states of being. I tend to resonate with the "state of being" theory. In 1963 the Catholic Church reversed its law governing cremation even though cremation is at odds with the resurrection of the body. We can believe whatever we want, but if we are alive in our human bodies right now, *we don't know*. We don't have any first-person experience.

As sugar maples grow older, they produce more flowers. After waiting thirty years to begin producing flowers, they flower only lightly at forty to sixty years of age. *It is not until the tree is seventy to one hundred years old that moderate flowering occurs.* Mom will be eighty in two days. She has reached her peak flowering. She has flowered longer than most of her family. All of nature is anchored in cycles related to timing. A sugar maple can live to be three hundred to four hundred years old. Mom never thought she would live to be eighty years old. But she has—or almost.

I think she would have died at age sixty had she not had open-heart surgery. These decisions are often made during a crisis when we are least able to think clearly and rationally. When faced with the imminent loss of someone we love, if given a chance for survival with a medical intervention, most of us will say yes. Mom said yes. We all said yes twenty years ago when the arteries feeding Mom's heart became clogged with cholesterol. While she has had many wonderful moments over the last twenty years, she has never returned to her baseline level of health. Side effects from the medications and other limitations started to show up with greater frequency after her surgery.

Maple decline is a term used to refer to maple trees suffering a variety of conditions. There is no consistent cause, but rather a combination of factors such as mechanical injury, weather stress, injury from road salts, planting too deeply, or nutrient imbalances. Once this condition sets in, it is easier for other pathogens to take advantage of the tree. The tips of the branches will begin to die. Enough leaves will drop to give the tree a scarce look, and a slow decline will take place over a number of years. *Mom has been suffering from maple decline.* It is easier in our culture to say yes than it is to say no. Families are often at odds, with these types of life-or-death decisions adding even more muddiness to an already complex issue.

The importance of these conversations happening before an emergency is one of the ways we can grow

Chapter Fourteen: Sugar Maple Tree

more clarity around this topic. Education is essential. We often put more time into learning how to do just about anything else *than we do into our own mortality.* I make a personal pledge to return home with a new awareness of the importance of these discussions around life and death with my husband and my daughter and her husband. Thank you, Mom, for continuing to be my teacher.

> **Journal entry November 13, 2020, 8:30 p.m.** *The way I am showing up present, thoughtful, and open is the way I want to show up for all of my life. With the same care I am taking during this time with Mom leaving her body. This moment is big, but does this moment demand any more or less care than every other moment?*

> **Journal entry November 14, 2020.** *Sitting here with Mom and my sisters. It is a beautiful sunny day. We had a service with Father Nick. Mom received last rites and we all took Communion. Mom said she feels blessed and free. She is so happy we took Communion with her. One day until November 15.*

Mom is sleeping in her bedroom. My sisters and I have quietly transformed the living room with strands of tiny glowing lights. An altar holds Paul's photo, our rosaries, Mom's beloved statue of Mother Mary, and some rose quartz. Rose quartz is known as the stone of unconditional love. Its energy is believed to release strong vibrations and increase feelings of peace and compassion. Also, on the altar is a beautiful floral head wreath that one of Mom's friends who is aware of her plan has made for her. We have little bits of Mom's favorite foods to nibble on.

When Mom wakes from her sleep, we bathe her. Like holy water washing her earthly film away, we let layers of life puddle around her pale, fragile, age-marked body. We handle her with care, as if she is breakable. We wash her hair using her favorite shampoo. We apply lotion to her well-worn skin. We do this quietly, not with sadness, but with reverence. *Our own version of last rites.* Does she know she is loved? Has our love been enough to fill her and prepare her for tomorrow?

Mom loves the transformation in the living room. We are making a memory. We nibble at the food. None of us are really hungry, but we are Italian; food

Chapter Fourteen: Sugar Maple Tree

is a cultural part of any important occasion. At 8:40 p.m., Mom is ready for bed. She encourages us to play Mexican Train Dominoes at the dining-room table. She wants her last night to be filled with the sounds of joy coming from all three of her daughters. We tuck her into bed and get out the dominoes. None of us were sure what we would be doing on Mom's last night on earth, but I can guarantee you we didn't think we would be playing dominoes. We check with Mom. "Are we too loud, Mom?" "No, girls. I love hearing your laughter."

Mom has been sleeping for some time now and we are about one hour into our game when my sister and I decide to smoke some hash. Because Mom has been on supplemental oxygen for years, we have not had candles in the house for a very long time. Hence, no lighters and no matches. I can only suppose it was our "Mom is dying tomorrow morning at 11:00 a.m. stupor" that has caused us to revert back to our teenage years. We retrieve two butter knives out of the drawer in the kitchen and proceed to hot knife the hash. All of a sudden, from Mom's room we hear "Girls, I smell smoke!" Looking at each other with wide eyes, we try to suppress our giggles. "It's OK, Mom. You go back to sleep. Everything is under control."

Our youngest sister won the game. I have the scores recorded in my journal. We have been taking turns sleeping with Mom, and tonight is not my turn. I want to sleep with Mom, but I also trust there is a larger divine plan always taking place, and tonight that plan has placed my middle sister with Mom. I head downstairs. It feels like sleep will evade me tonight, but I fall asleep shortly after my head hits the pillow. Tomorrow is November 15. *Ten more hours until Mom leaves.*

Today is November 15. Mom's eightieth birthday. I awaken to the faint sounds of movement upstairs. Looking at the clock, I am surprised to see one hand pointed at the eight and the other at the twelve. Have I managed to sleep for eight hours? Alone in the bed, I give myself a few more minutes nestled into the warm covers. "*Please, God, hold us up today as we say goodbye to our mother. Greet her with your white light and open arms. Mary, if you are around, I am sure Mom would love to meet you in person. She has been talking to you for most of her life. Amen.*"

Chapter Fourteen: Sugar Maple Tree

Arriving upstairs, I find Mom and my sister in the kitchen. "What are you guys doing?" I ask. My sister informs me that they are "baking shortbread." Both Mom and my sister look a bit disheveled, and that matches the countertop and floor, which are both wearing a soft coat of white flour. "Really ... shortbread?" "Yes," my sister replies. "I am making Mom a shortbread birthday cake using her recipe." This is not how I thought we would start this day, but apparently shortbread is now part of the protocol, along with George Harrison and maple leaves. This sister is the daughter who carries on Mom's tradition of baking. We all look forward to her lavish and overflowing Christmas cookie trays. Her monster chocolate chip cookies and her butter tarts filled with gooey brown sugar and juicy plump raisins are coveted by all of us.

At some point she realized the shortbread mixture was too dry and too crumbly, and that is when she decided to enlist Mom's help. She quietly tiptoed into the bedroom, not wanting to wake our other sister, who had crawled into bed with them in the wee hours of the morning.

"Mom... Mom. I am so sorry to wake you so early on the day of your dying, but I can't get the shortbread right. It's too crumbly." Mom stirs and opens her eyes. Half asleep, she mumbles "What?" "I'm sorry, Mom, but I really need your help. I wouldn't ask, but after today you can sleep for a really long, long time." Mom's eyes take in my sisters. "Mother Mary pin a rose on me ... I'm getting up. I can't believe I am getting up on the day I am dying to make my own birthday cake!"

My sister helped Mom into the kitchen with her walker and oxygen in tow. Mom looked at the bowl. "What is this?" she asked with a mixture of confusion and slight impatience. "I don't know, Mom. I followed the recipe to a T." "Well, it doesn't look right," she replied. "It's too dry." They looked at the recipe Mom had written out in her shaky cursive. One of the remnants of Mom's fifth-grade education is her unique spelling. She spells everything phonetically. Sugar might be spelled *shugir*. It was an ongoing joke between us girls. Mom's spelling. Mom looked at the recipe. "Well, I can see this isn't written right." To which my sister replied, "I'm glad we figured this out now, Mom. I could have been following this recipe for the rest of my life wondering what I was screwing up!" They proceeded to

Chapter Fourteen: Sugar Maple Tree

remedy the mixture, and the shortbread went into the oven to bake.

Mom asked my sister to help her clean up and dress. She has chosen a simple white linen tunic to wear on her last day. She brushed her teeth. She combed her hair and we placed the flower wreath on Mom's head. When my youngest sister and I came up dressed in our silky cream-colored PJ Harlow pajamas, our "Oprah" pajamas, as they had once been one of *"Oprah's favorite things,"* our middle sister looked at the two of us. "Apparently I didn't get the memo about the dress code." "What dress code?" we answered sheepishly.

Our youngest sister's husband is here with us. For thirty-eight years he has sometimes begrudgingly but always without fail run errands for Mom when we were not available. He has taken her to doctor appointments. He has brought what she needed and forgot to bring to her frequent hospitalizations. He has bought her groceries. He has shown up. For a guy who did not grow up in a large close family like ours, he has often found all of us a bit overwhelming. He's a solitary guy, much like my own husband. During the last three months, he and

Mom have healed years of angst just by showing up authentically. Love, love, and more love. It is right that he is here with us.

As our sister carried in the shortbread cake with candles lit, I wondered if the combination of the lit candles and Mom's oxygen compressor would blow the whole house up and we wouldn't have to go through with MAID. We sing a half-hearted happy birthday and take some photos. We are sitting with Mom. The atmosphere is somber. All we have to do is continue breathing and stay present. The rap at the door came around 9:45 a.m. The nurse is early. She offers to leave and come back, but Mom has thrust her arm out and said, "Now is as good a time as any." *Mom is ready.* The nurse is kind and soft-spoken and skilled at inserting IV catheters. I am grateful she gets it in one stick. We give her a piece of shortbread.

The next tap at the door is the physician. He enters quietly and his gaze takes in the living room, the altar, the twinkling lights, Mom's wreath of flowers. He looks at us. "This is beautiful. You girls have done well. Daughters are great. With sons, they often sit on the couch in the living room while I

Chapter Fourteen: Sugar Maple Tree

administer the medication to the family member in the bedroom." We have done our best. There is no right way. The MAID handbook does not teach you how to show up. We have created a ceremony the way Mom has taught us to create ceremonies for any special event. *We are making a memory.*

Before the physician arrived, we had made up Mom's bed. We placed her meaningful treasures on her dresser so she could see them. The sweet birch tree with tiny twinkling lights that Paul's son had given his Grams for her birthday. Mom's statue of Mother Mary. Paul's photo. Rose quartz. The essence of lavender from the diffuser is filling the room with a soft, sweet, floral scent. "My Sweet Lord" is queued up. George Harrison, the quiet Beatle, will sing Mom out on her journey. On Mom's wrist she is wearing our three moonstone bracelets. We hope she can infuse them with enough love to carry us through this moment and the days to come.

Mom lay down, and like kittens we lay down beside her and tucked ourselves in. The nurse started the music. The doctor asked Mom, "Do you wish to continue?" Mom answered "Yes." As he administers the medication I start to say, "Fly to the light, Mom…"

but she is already on her way. She whispers "shhh-hhhhhh," and quietly, peacefully, silently her spirit left her body. Mom had asked us to please leave the room if we felt like we were going to fall apart at any time, but we didn't. We didn't fall apart. Instead, we fell *into* the magic and mystery of what was happening. Our tears were silent tears. Nobody spoke. The doctor and the nurse had quietly slipped out and made their departure.

Chapter Fourteen: Sugar Maple Tree

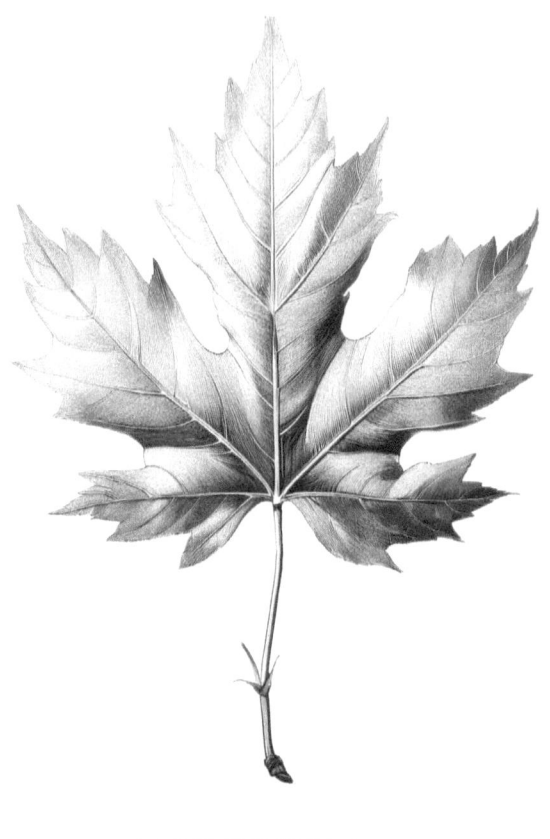

Acer saccharum leaf
Common Name – Sugar Maple leaf

Palmate leaves resemble an open hand. Their five lobes radiate from a single point and mimic our five fingers. Whenever I am in Mom's kitchen, this tree lures me in with its beauty. Thousands of hands masquerading as leaves are energetically holding us up with quiet strength.

Chapter Fifteen

Fly to the Light

Journal entry November 15, 2020. *We lay with Mom for what felt like hours. Soaking in the moment. Letting it leave its imprint on our hearts, our minds, our cells, our spirits. In the past, when I have told this story I would say we lay with Mom for two hours. My sisters have corrected me. Apparently, it was more like thirty minutes. Time had slowed for me. We all got up at once. My sister's dog Gaia, whom Mom had helped to raise, took her spot at the top of Mom's head and would not move again until Mom's body was removed.*

We walked into the kitchen and looked at each other. Our tear-streaked faces serene. We had done it. We had showed up and held Mom as she took flight. It felt right. We all decided we were not ready to part with Mom just yet. We called family to let them know that Mom was gone. That she had departed quietly. We cleaned up the kitchen. We ate a piece of shortbread. We walked around in circles. We didn't try to fill the space with words. The space was already filled with love.

At 2:00 p.m. we decided we were ready to let Mom's body go. We called the funeral home and told the exceptional funeral director that he could come and pick Mom up. He arrived quickly. We removed our bracelets from Mom's wrist and placed them on our own wrists. They placed Mom in a dark green canvas bag with a cross appliqued on the top. I didn't see it. My sister said she didn't like it. Mom wanted to be carried out in her own blanket, but that was not practical. There really is truth to the phrase dead weight.

At the precise moment they opened the back door to Mom's porch and began to carry her down the stairs, the stillness of the day was interrupted by a strong gust of wind that swept through and removed almost every remaining leaf on the sugar maple tree. A large branch split and hit the ground. Mom was gone.

The term "wake" is thought to have come from the practice of mourners keeping vigil over the dead body all through the night until it is buried. In place of sleep, we stay a-wake. The body is never left alone to protect it from mischievous spirits and demons that might wish to cause harm or steal the

Chapter Fifteen: Fly to the Light

soul. Clocks are stopped at the time of death to fool the spirits, and mirrors are covered or turned, lest they provide a portal to other worlds. This is a time for everyone to come and place their hands on the body, kiss their loved one or friend goodbye, tell stories about the deceased, and mourn and celebrate with both laughter and tears.

If we were having a traditional Irish wake, Mom's body would still be with us—in her home until we followed it to the crematorium. In some traditions, that is three full days. Time for the spirit or soul to completely leave the body and travel to heaven. Culturally, we have grown a lot of fear around death. People can go most of their lives without seeing or touching a dead body. This fear is often a reflection of how we feel about our own mortality. *If it is possible for someone else to die, that means I can die too.* Death often happens in hospitals and not in our homes with family holding vigil. As a nurse, I witnessed death on a regular basis—especially in the critical care units. It was a privilege for me to be with people when they were leaving their bodies.

I learned not to fear death from Mom. She attended many deaths as a caregiver. On the very first day of Mom's very first job as a nurse's aide, she walked into her very first room and came face to face with her *very first dead body*. Mom told me the resident was sitting up, as if to eat breakfast, but she was dead. Mom went out and told the head nurse, who replied, "I was just in there and sat her up for breakfast. Go back in and make sure she's really dead. She's probably just sleeping." Mom returned to the room and looked closely. She looked dead. She lay her head tentatively on the woman's chest. No heartbeat. She held her trembling hand under the woman's nostrils. No breath. Mom went back out. "I think she really is dead."

Even though Mom's body is now lying in the funeral home, we will honor our Irish heritage with our version of a wake this evening. Right now, Mom's death is a closely guarded secret to all but a few. My sisters and I can complete this part of the journey with Mom and with each other without distraction. My sisters set about cleaning the house and preparing the space and sent me off to the market for food and libations. This would be a double ceremony—Mom's wake and her eightieth birthday. We had learned about ceremony from Mom. Dress is important and requires some thought.

Chapter Fifteen: Fly to the Light

We decided we would bring Mom to the party by wearing her clothes. In Mom's bedroom, we opened her closets. There were all of Mom's clothes. All of her favorite colors. Pastel pinks and yellows. Light blues, periwinkles, and soft yellow-greens. Lots of scarves. Mom loved scarves. I would choose one to bring home for Stephanie. Most of these clothes had been gifts from her daughters. Given with love over many years and many birthdays. We started taking clothes out of the closet. Mom's scent had taken up residence in the linen and cotton fibers. It intermingled with the lavender still carried in the air from this morning. Gaia had resumed her vigil and curled into a ball on Mom's pillow. I felt a twinge of jealousy. Like she was still communicating with Mom in a way I couldn't. We were on a mission. Each of us looking for the perfect outfit to wear to the party. Like three teenage girls dressing for a big date, we proceeded to try on almost all of the clothes in Mom's closets. Tossing aside tops and pants and skirts and dresses we decided didn't work, we continued to empty Mom's closets until eventually, we each stood in our perfect *Mom outfit*.

We left the bedroom and headed for the living room. It seemed fitting that we should start Mom's wake with the Rosary. We took our rosaries off from around our necks. At this time, I think the rosary felt like the lifeline Mom had said it would. Our connection with the other side. We knelt in front of the altar we had created for Mom. I began, "Hail Mary, full of grace, the Lord is with thee. Blessed art thou amongst women, and blessed is the fruit of thy womb, Jesus."

My sisters responded, "Holy Mary, Mother of God. Pray for us sinners, now and at the hour of our death. Amen."

And we fell back into the call and return cadence we had intoned so often as children. My sister describes this night as *"The best night of my life."* We sang. We drummed. We played Mexican Train Dominoes. We ate. We drank. We cried. We laughed. We celebrated each other and we celebrated Mom. We were still under the spell that had been cast that morning. Ordinary life had yet to disrupt our rhapsody. *We still had a minute.*

Journal entry November 18, 2020. Such a whirlwind since you left, Mom. We thought we were prepared, but every day there are a hundred unimportant details that require

Chapter Fifteen: Fly to the Light

our attention. It has been three days. Seventy-two hours. Four thousand three hundred and twenty minutes since November 15. When you said, "The pain of my leaving is going to stop you girls in your tracks and drop you to your knees," I thought you were exaggerating, but my knees feel bruised, Mom. You knew it would be like this because this is how you felt when Paul died, isn't it? Now I know your grief. Paul was one of your branches. You weren't exaggerating either. I dropped to my knees when I walked into the funeral home and looked at you the morning after your spirit took flight. I stumbled to your body and all but laid myself on top of you, longing to draw anything that was left of you into me. I know I was not hugging my mother. I gave your cold waxy forehead one last kiss and stepped back. Disintegration and integration. It was clear you were gone, and despite the depth of my grief, I still felt you had made the right decision for you.

Now I understand why the exceptional funeral director suggested we get at least a dozen death certificates. Each death certificate releases us from an obligation that shackles us to Mom's earthly life, when all we want right now is to be tethered to her heavenly spirit life. The sugar maple tree in the back yard is bare. Just three days ago it was still full of golden palmate leaves. Their lobes or fingers had dried and curled at the tips as the trunk was preparing for winter by commandeering all of the tree's energy into the root system.

My sisters are still talking about the thousands of maple leaves that flew off the multibranched limbs when they carried Mom's body out the door. It was as if they had waited to be tossed from the branches so they could escort Mom on her journey. I wish I had been there to witness that moment. I think I was doing some ordinary task like using the restroom. *This is grieving.* Learning how to integrate our laid-bare hearts with the ordinary tasks that still require our attention. I wonder, "Where did those leaves carry my mom?" I don't feel anxious about it, just curious. Was it simply a matter of letting go? From my perspective, it looked like Mom simply lost consciousness, but I'm asking about what happened after that. *That which we cannot see...*

With deciduous trees, a hormone communicates a chemical message to the leaves that it is time to

Chapter Fifteen: Fly to the Light

leave the branch. I know the physiological processes that happen when we die. Cell membranes disintegrate and release enzymes that begin auto-digestion. With maple leaves, abscission cells converge where the stem meets the branch. Like microscopic scissors, they cut the leaf away from the mother tree. Leaves don't drop from trees. They are actually cut away from the branch. We are like three leaves that have been cut from the mother tree. But in our case, the mother tree has left the leaves. It will be some time before we find our new landing place.

My strong suit has always been efficiency. I once had a boss who described my proclivity for productivity by stating, "Ask Theresa to cook your breakfast, and she will build you a pancake house by the end of the day." While they say it is impossible to actually multitask, I have done a fairly good job of faking it for most of my life. *I sense there is nothing efficient about grief and mourning.* If any multitasking is to occur, it will focus on how to show up for life when waves of sensations come like thieves to steal my breath away.

Does the mother tree feel pain when a branch breaks off? Science says trees do not have brains, nervous systems, or pain receptors, and therefore they are not capable of feeling pain. Humans, on the other hand, come with rich sensory and motor nervous systems through which we are constantly responding to the world around us. We have worked tirelessly to finish preparing the house and tying up the loose ends. It is good to have something to keep us busy and distract our hearts.

Breath by breath we are integrating the reality that Mom is truly gone. The sensations come in waves. Like water lapping onto the shores of my beloved Lake Michigan. Every once in a while, and usually without warning, a large wave rolls in and tumbles my heart. Like a beach stone being carried under by the current, I know from experience the best way to deal with a riptide is to stay calm and relaxed while swimming parallel to the shore until you can get back. With each moment that passes, my longing to be home grows stronger. I miss Pete. I miss Stephanie. I miss my dogs Lucy and Lily.

It has been just over three and a half months since I left home, but I don't want to leave my sisters too soon. I have kept my promise to Mom, and I have stayed until it feels like they are ready for me to go. Today is Wednesday. We have most of the house

Chapter Fifteen: Fly to the Light

stuff taken care of. Wesley is now in possession of the rest of Mom's home goods and furniture. The girls will take care of the clothes and finish settling the estate. Tomorrow I will take my tender heart and my exhausted body home. It feels right. It's time.

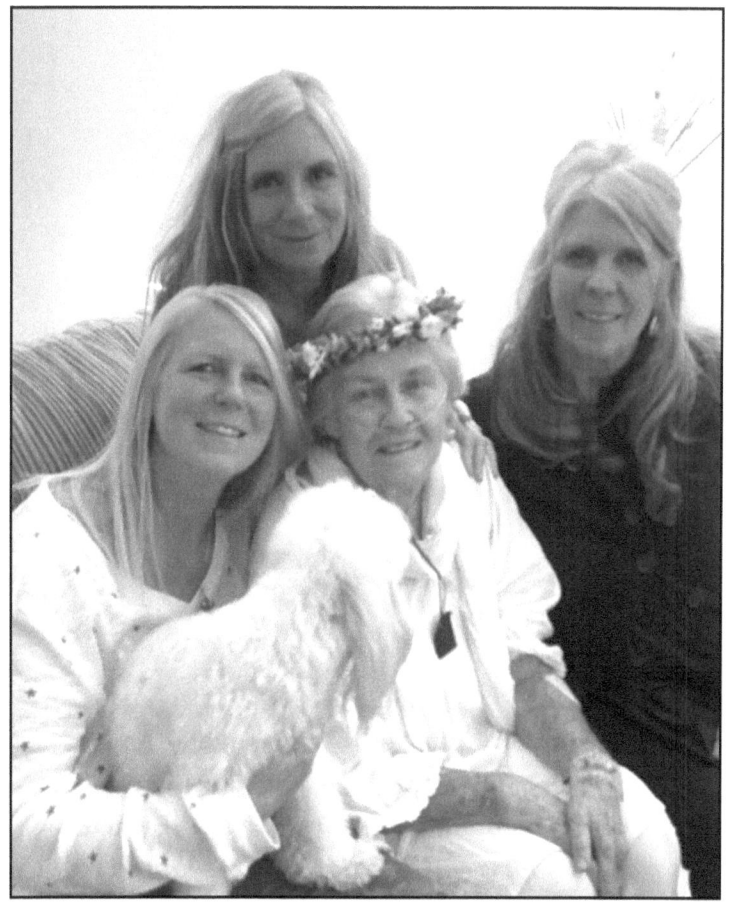

Making a memory. We took this photo one hour before mom died.

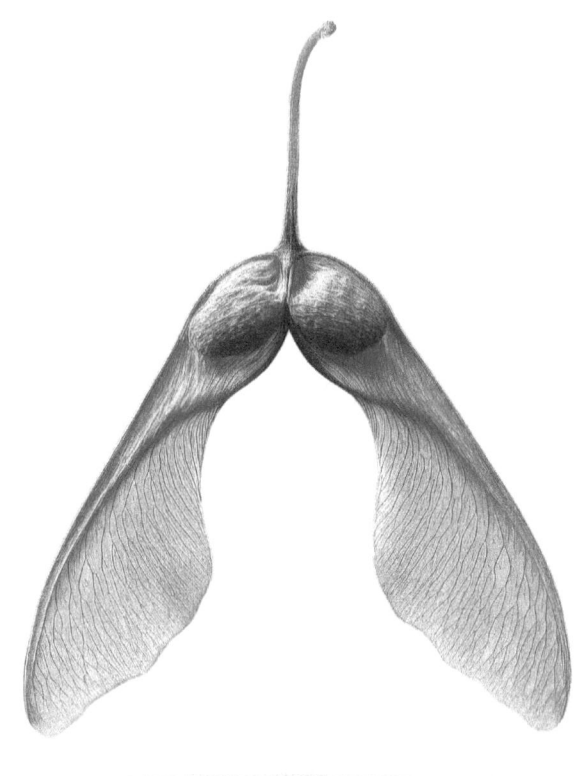

Samara
Common Name – Keys or helicopters

These winged seeds let the autumn winds guide them to an arbitrary landing place. A potential place to support the DNA program of the seed and germinate a new plant, or a place to decompose.

Epilogue

GRIEF

Dear Mom,

I remember the first Sunday after you left. I had been home for three days. I lay on the couch and covered myself with my favorite well-loved blanket. Pete tucked me in like you had when I was a young child. Thank you for all of those "tuck-ins," Mom. Thank you for washing and drying the essence of nature into my fresh-off-the-line sheets. I will feel you in nature and I will smell you in line-dried sheets. I let the weighted blanket anchor me. I felt myself slowly pour out a weariness that had gradually oozed into my cells as I said goodbye to your earthly presence.

I was practicing the value of resilience you had imprinted on me. I felt the depth of my fatigue, and little by little I began to soften. It was erratic at first and shaky, like the somatic experience of releasing long-held tension. Lucy and Lily sensed my fatigue and became two dog sentries standing guard. One at my head and one at my feet; two furry blankets had welcomed me home with their unconditional love and devotion. I sank into a bottomless deep sleep for hours. There were tears and I remember keening for you like a kitten mewling for its mother. Was I awake or was I dreaming? It had felt like both. It could have been either. My most vivid recollection that afternoon was of not feeling you. It seemed you were entirely, completely gone.

The ache that had settled into my heart with your leaving was soothed only by a deeper knowing that all was well. This was grief. I needed a long rest and the quiet and solitude of winter days. I needed to feel all of the sensations. I decided then to embrace the quality of time that was the "after."

Our raspberry bushes have outgrown their space. They are competing with some well-established northern white cedars for the sun, and the cedars are winning. I remember that Mom told me raspberry bushes love to drink in six to eight hours of full sun each day. Like most things, they can tolerate less, but that results in fewer berries. That was me when I returned home after Mom's body died. It was the end of November and the cold had finally set in. With shorter and cooler days, the plants

Epilogue: Grief

had started diverting their remaining sap to their roots. This last sap is nature's antifreeze. The plants' cells were sending their water down to the roots in a process called hardening. Like a plant acclimating to its new environment, I was acclimating to life without my mom. My vitality, my creativity, my spontaneity, my ability to grow new fruit had hardened. I was relying on the reserves in my roots to carry me through the grieving period. In plant language, it was time to close my stomata and limit transpiration. I needed to conserve water.

How do you reenter everyday life after such a profound experience? I had searched my consciousness for the instruction manual, but it was not to be found. Tradition can help navigate us at a time when it would be so easy to drive right off the road, or never even start the car. If we were in Italy, I might have spent my days baking ossa di morti, "bones of the dead" cookies. I created my own mourning rituals. Altars appeared all over our home. I brought up three fallen birch trees from the woods whose height spanned floor to ceiling and turned a corner of the dining room into a forest. I filled our house with nature. It was the healing balm I craved then and the balm that continues to soothe me now.

I placed Mom's rhubarb steppingstones in a circle around the trees. Their branches held tiny fairy lights that mimicked fireflies and illuminated the corner. Photos, crystals, fossils, and anything else that felt sacred appeared on my altars. Feathers, dimes, Mom's medicine pouch, her diamond bracelet and Reiki crystal all lived on the altars. Pete understood my need to mourn in this way and he helped me arrange the rhubarb leaves around the birch trees.

Journal entry December 3, 2020. It feels like time is shape-shifting. Even writing feels like too much work. You flew away eighteen days ago. Eighteen days feels like eighteen minutes, feels like eighteen years, feels like eighteen seconds.

I sent a newsletter to my students.

"It's been eighteen days since my mom's body died. I don't for a minute feel or think the essence that is my mom died. But something died … for sure. I was there. I saw it and I felt it. When I look up 'death' in the dictionary, one definition is 'the permanent ending of vital processes in a cell or tissue.' That, I believe is true. Her

Epilogue: Grief

body died. The rest of her took flight. The pang of loss comes for me when I realize there is space now where her physical presence is gone.

"I will miss the almost daily conversations we had as I described my adventures while traveling for work, and Mom described her adventures while working on her next painting or in her garden. Several times a day water will begin to spill out of my eyes as somatically I feel the huge shift that has occurred. I really understand 'somatic cringing' now. It arises involuntarily, when I remember at a cellular and energetic level the profound impact of our relationship on my life. I don't want these tears to go away until I have completely known the depth of the sensations.

"There are moments when I feel stopped in my tracks, and that is when my husband or daughter will wrap their arms around me and I can sink into their safety nets. A greater loss for me would be forgetting the feeling of love my mom and I had for each other. That love kept us connected even during those times we weren't sure we even liked each other."

✧✧✧

I remember feeling that nothing would ever be the same for me. Groceries, cooking, laundry, cleaning, dog walking, correspondence, paying bills, and all of the activities that asked me to show up had not stopped when Mom died. They continued as if the world had absolutely no understanding of the profound and life-altering event I had just taken part in. They felt like impositions, when walking, rock hounding, creating altars and shrines, swinging, journaling, movement and music were the activities I needed to soothe my aching heart. To say goodbye. To prepare for spring.

Hiking the forest with Lucy and Lily, I could hide my tender heart and be the introvert I needed to be. Talking took too much focus. Too much energy. When we stepped under the hobbit-like stone arch constructed of large chunks of dolomite and limestone, my grief felt safe. My breath would begin to match the cadence of my steps that had walked this trail on this end of the Niagara Escarpment for twenty years now. In the summer I walked barefoot on the carpet of dry pine needles lining the forest floor. In the winter I skied. Sometimes I ran. Traversing Hotz Trail past Europe Lake and through Newport State

Epilogue: Grief

Park became my version of going to church. A cathedral where the choir wears speckled wings.

Dear Mom,

How many years did I walk this trail talking to you on the phone? The last two years we used Facetime so you could walk with me and see what I saw. We had walked in every season.

We still walk together, but it's different. I still have a close relationship with you. I talk to you daily. I still seek your advice, and I have learned to be patient and wait for your answer. It's like learning a new language at first. Sometimes an overwhelming longing for your earthly presence will rise from the depth of my heart. Tears will surface as a tangible container for my grief. These moments stop me in my tracks. I don't want to miss any of them. I love this experience that still connects me to the depth of our relationship.

Early on when I was still racked with grief, your presence was not clear to me. The physical, mental, and emotional toll of acute grief drained me and took most of my energy. But you leaving your body was about what was right for you. My grief is about me.

There is that which we can see and that which we cannot see.... I wear the rosary you gave me hidden under my shirt. I haven't been able to take it off yet. The pads of my fingers are memorizing the facets of the crystal beads. Lines from a poem I wrote years ago surface in my memory...

The sin that I confess to thee is sometimes walking thoughtlessly,
   but gentle breezes cleanse my soul,
   my eyes wide open makes me whole.
   Amid the choir's joyous sound,
   I bow to thee on sacred ground.

Author's Note

It has been almost five years since my mother died via MAID. There are times when I still miss her earthly presence—usually when I am grappling with some bit of life that would benefit from her motherly advice. There has not been one moment when I feel that she made the wrong decision by choosing MAID. I have shared her story with many people. While there have been a few who objected and one person whom I watched physically recoil—the overwhelming majority state their support for legalizing MAID or some form of assisted death in the United States.

As of this writing, Medical Assistance in Dying (MAID) is legal in eleven states and Washington, D.C. Eighteen states are in the process of considering some form of legislation supporting MAID. Labor pains are inevitable whenever we are birthing something new. The higher the stakes, the greater the labor pains. Most would agree that dying is a high-stakes act. I hope this book will provide a window into the experience of supporting someone who is transitioning out of their physical body regardless of the path they choose.

While my mom chose MAID, there are many ways to die. For most of us, I suspect there will come a time when we will be called to show up for a loved one who is dying. All of us will one day die ourselves. The world does not stop for these occasions, and they often happen in the midst of our already full lives. Discussions and advance planning can be helpful in mitigating the competing and complex moments that arise in the midst of death. Having these important conversations in advance can free us to be more present for those who are leaving by not making monumental decisions in the midst of great emotional and mental stress.

Canada allows a physician to administer the medications that will end a human life. They continue to use research-based evidence to grow the program and increase its availability for all eligible Canadians.

The United States has some of the most restrictive laws in the world around MAID. One must be able to ingest the medication on their own. This can be very stressful for all involved. What if the person

AUTHOR'S NOTE

can't swallow? What if they vomit back the medication? What if a neurodegenerative disease prevents self-administration? What if they lapse into a coma and don't die? I am grateful Mom did not have to open capsules and consume a bitter concoction that can take some time to work if you even manage to swallow it.

While conversations are taking place around self-administration versus clinician administered assisted death, there remains a lot of controversy and gray areas in the laws governing assisted death in the United States. If we want to have a say, we need to speak up and make ourselves heard. Please stay informed and check your sources. There is a lot of false information circulating about MAID, and the truth is readily available. Following are resources that I found helpful while writing *Choosing to Die*.

Choosing to die

RESOURCES

Government of Canada
Medical Assistance in Dying
https://www.canada.ca/en/health-canada/services/health-services-benefits/medical-assistance-dying.html#a1

Compassion & Choices
8156 S. Wadsworth Blvd #E-162
Littleton, CO 80128
https://compassionandchoices.org

Death with Dignity
PO Box 2009
Portland, OR 97208
https://deathwithdignity.org

National Institutes of Health (NIH)
Study: "Rethinking Medical Aid in Dying"
https://pmc.ncbi.nlm.nih.gov/articles/PMC10258856/

Books

The Day I Die: The Untold Story of Assisted Dying in America
by Anita Hannig

The Last Doctor
by Dr. Jean Marmoreo and Johanna Schneller

In My Time of Dying
by Sebastian Junger

Being Mortal
by Atul Gawande

Briefly Perfectly Human
by Alua Arthur

In Love: A Memoir of Love and Loss
by Amy Bloom

This Is Assisted Dying: A Doctor's Story of Empowering Patients at the End of Life
by Stefanie Green, MD

Acknowledgments

Several years ago while I was still teaching, a participant in the workshop walked up to me at the end of the weekend and handed me her business card. That was Bethany Kelly, founder of Publishing Partner, a company that helps independent authors publish their books. I hung on to the card, and when I started to write *Choosing to Die,* I pulled that card out of my desk and contacted Bethany for advice. She has been a guiding light for me during this entire process. I am forever grateful for Bethany's skills, expertise, encouragement, and support.

Anaik, your developmental edit has been invaluable. Your suggestions allowed me to tell my story with greater clarity and flow. You challenged me to hone my writing skills, and in doing so I became a better writer. You will be my editor for life.

Frank, thank you for your attention to detail, made softer by your sense of humor. I will rely on you to cross my "t's" and dot my "i's" from here on out.

Stefan, I tried to imagine what the "container" might look like to hold my words. Your skills exceeded what I could imagine. Thank you for the beautiful design you have created.

Steve and Debbie, thank you for the botanical illustrations you both created. They add dimension and grace to the writing. I know Mom would love them.

Wendy Andrews convinced me she could take a beautiful photograph of me that would complement my writing, and I think she did. Thank you, Wendy!

Thank you to Sara, Mel, Karen, and Debbie, who read and reread chapters for me over the past two years. Your feedback has kept propelling me forward.

Thank you, sisters. You lived this journey with me. We walked with grace, and when we tripped and fell, we picked each other up. I love you both dearly.

Thank you, Pete, for forty years of unwavering support and love.

Glossary

Annual: A plant that completes its life cycle, from germination to the production of seeds, within one growing season, and then dies.

Apex: The apex of a plant refers to the tip or highest point of an element, such as a stem or leaf. Specifically, the shoot apex is the growing tip of the stem, while the root apex is the tip of the root. These apices contain tissue responsible for plant growth. The term "apex" can also refer to the tip of other plant parts, like leaves or petals.

Autotrophic: A plant that can produce its own food through a process called photosynthesis.

Biennial: A flowering plant that, generally in a temperate climate, takes two years to complete its biological life cycle.

Corm: A specialized, swollen underground plant stem that acts as a storage organ, providing nutrients for the plant's growth and survival.

Corolla: The petals of a flower as a group, typically forming a whorl within the sepals and enclosing the reproductive organs.

Deadhead: In gardening, this refers to the process of removing faded or spent flowers from plants. This practice encourages the plant to redirect its energy toward producing new blooms and overall growth, rather than focusing on seed production. It also helps maintain a tidy appearance in the garden.

Dichogamous: Plants whose male and female reproductive organs (stamens and pistils, respectively) mature at different times. This temporal separation is a strategy to promote cross-pollination and prevent self-pollination.

Disc floret: In plants, disc florets are small, tubular flowers that form the central part of the flower head, also known as the capitulum or head. Disc florets are typically found in the center of the flower head.

First-order vein: In plant anatomy, "first-order vein" refers to the main or primary veins that run from the base of the leaf to the tip, often called the midrib. These are the largest and most prominent veins in a leaf, branching off into smaller veins of subsequent orders.

Heliotropic: Plants that exhibit heliotropism, a behavior where they turn their leaves or flowers to follow the sun's apparent movement across the sky.

Herbaceous plants: Non-woody plants, characterized by soft green stems that lack the persistent woody tissue found in trees and shrubs. They typically die back to the ground each year, either entirely (annuals and biennials) or partially (perennials), with new growth emerging from the base or underground parts the following season.

Heterotrophic: A plant that cannot produce its own food through photosynthesis and therefore relies on other organisms for nutrients.

Inflorescence: The complete flower head of a plant, including stems, stalks, bracts, and flowers.

Glossary

Krebs cycle: The Krebs cycle, also known as the citric acid cycle or tricarboxylic acid (TCA) cycle, is a series of chemical reactions that extract energy from molecules, particularly those derived from carbohydrates, fats, and proteins. It is the sequence of reactions by which most living cells generate energy during the process of aerobic respiration.

Node: In plant biology, a node is a point on a plant's stem where leaves, branches, or aerial roots grow from.

Panicle: A type of branched flower cluster, or inflorescence.

Peltate: In botany, peltate describes a leaf or other structure where the petiole (stalk) is attached to the underside of the blade (the flat part of the leaf), not at the base or margin. This gives the leaf a shield-like or umbrella-like appearance.

Perennial: A plant that lives for more than two years, often returning season after season.

Petiole: The stalk that supports a leaf and attaches it to the stem of a plant. It acts as a bridge, connecting the leaf blade to the main plant body.

Photosynthesis: The process by which plants, algae, and some bacteria convert light energy into chemical energy, creating sugars and releasing oxygen.

Phototropism: The growth or turning of a plant in response to a light stimulus.

Pistils: The female organs of a flower, comprising the stigma, style, and ovary.

Pollen: A fine, powdery substance produced by flowering plants for reproduction. It contains the male reproductive cells, which are transferred to the female part of the plant, either by wind, water, or animals (pollinators), to enable fertilization and seed production.

Ray floret: The petal-like structures surrounding the disc florets. Ray florets are found on the periphery.

Rhizome: A plant rhizome is a modified stem, typically growing horizontally either at or just below the soil surface, that produces roots and shoots from its nodes.

Root rot: A plant disease characterized by the decay and deterioration of a plant's root system, often caused by excessive moisture or certain fungi.

Rosette: A plant whose leaves grow in a circular, radiating pattern, resembling a rose. This growth pattern is characterized by leaves that cluster tightly together, either at the base of the plant (basal rosette) or at the end of stems.

Samara: A type of dry, one-seeded fruit characterized by a flattened, wing-like structure that develops from the ovary wall. It is found in trees such as maple, ash, elm, and sycamore. The unique shape of the samara allows it to spin like a helicopter's rotor when falling, enabling the wind to carry the seed away from the parent plant, aiding in seed dispersal.

Sepal: The sepal is the outer part of a flower that encloses and protects the developing bud. Collectively, sepals form the calyx. They are usually green and lie underneath the more colorful petals when the flower is open.

Glossary

Stamen: The male fertilizing organ of a flower, typically consisting of a pollen-containing anther and a filament.

Stomata: Tiny pores, or openings, typically found on the surface of leaves, stems, and other plant parts. They are crucial for gas exchange, allowing plants to take in carbon dioxide for photosynthesis and release oxygen.

Thigmotropism: A plant's directional growth response to touch or physical contact with a solid object. This response is typically characterized by a bending or coiling of plant parts, like tendrils, as they grow around a support.

Transpiration: The process where water evaporates from a plant's surface, primarily through tiny pores called stomata on leaves. This evaporation helps transport water and nutrients from the roots to the shoots and also plays a role in cooling the plant.

Trichomes: Hairlike outgrowths or appendages found on the surface of many plants. They are not just superficial structures; they play a crucial role in plant defense and survival by producing compounds that deter pests, protect against environmental stress, and even contribute to the plant's medicinal properties.

Umbel: An umbel is a type of flower cluster where several individual flower stalks (pedicels) radiate from a common point, resembling the ribs of an umbrella.

Choosing to die

ABOUT THE AUTHOR

Theresa E. Evans earned a Bachelor of Science degree in Nursing from Ball State University in 1992. Her nursing career spanned fifteen years with a focus in Critical and Cardiac Care. In 2007 Theresa opened Stone Path Yoga Studio after completing all levels of Critical Alignment Yoga Therapy and the requirements for the 500-hour Yoga Certification (RYT500). She is a Certified Clinical Somatic Educator who has taught workshops, Certified Trainings, classes, and private clients around the world how to move with less pain and more freedom. In her free time, she loves to putter in her garden with her husband, fossil hunt with her daughter, hike with her dogs, and write. She would describe herself as a *"freedom cultivator."*

CHOOSING TO DIE

www.ingramcontent.com/pod-product-compliance
Lightning Source LLC
LaVergne TN
LVHW091719070526
838199LV00050B/2462